5K

Fitness Run

By

David Holt

Author of:
Best Marathons
Running Dialogue
Best Half-Marathons
10K & 5K Running, Training & Racing

Cover pictures are the start of Santa Barbara's evening 5K race series. For 18 weeks, 15 to 45 minute 5K runners, plus walkers, enjoy a post race dinner with live music.

NOTE
The information in this book is not a substitute for professional fitness or medical advice. As with all self-improvement and exercise programs, seek medical approval before you begin running or other training and if discomfort occurs during or after exercise.

First Printing, July 2,004
Paperback ISBN # 0-9658897-5-0
Printing History   10 9 8 7 6 5 4 3 2 1

CONTENTS   page

Special thanks to the Portsmouth, Yeovil, Ventura and Santa Barbara running communities. Thanks for inspiration from Roy Benson, Bill Bowerman, Percy Cerutty, David Costell Ph.D. Jack Daniels Ph.D. Weldermar Gerschler, Gary N. Guten, Frank Horwill, Mihaly Igloe, Author Lydiard, Tim Noakes, Bruce Tulloh and Harry Wilson.

Books printed on paper by David Holt include:

Running Dialogue, 5K to the Marathon, 280 pages. ISBN # 0-9658897-4-2 $17.95. An excellent first book for beginners or an addition to your library for all athletes.

10K & 5K Running, Training & Racing: *The Running Pyramid*, 180 pages ISBN # 0-9658897-1-8 $17.95. Five training phases at 20 to 100 miles per week. Low intensity 20 mile per week runners enjoy the science and running techniques just as much as the 60 mile per week runners.

Best Half Marathons: *Jog, Run, Train or Walk & Race the Half Marathon.*   224 pages   ISBN # 0-9658897-6-9 $17.95. Graduate from 10K training with the half-marathon. Extensive cross training & schedules for half marathon to 20 mile racing for joggers and elite runners.

Best Marathons: *Jog, Run, Train or Walk & Race your First Marathon or Fast Marathons.* 396 pages   ISBN # 0-9658897-0-X $17.95.   Five training phases totaling 10 to 50 weeks to your marathon, plus extensive nutrition and injury advice.

(In 2,005) *5K Fitness Walk*, at $14.95 includes extensive nutrition advice and walking to beat more than 20 diseases.

This book is *5K Fitness Run* ISBN # 0-9658897-5-0 230 pages at $14.95 Healthy beginnings to 5K races at 12-30 miles per week.

Order these paperback books from any main street or Internet bookstore, or see page 240 to get signed copies, direct from him. Most are also available as e-books.

Introduction

According to the Surgeon General, with regular exercise, you can avoid being one of the quarter of a million people each year who commit suicide from the lack of exercise.

The 5K (a mere 3 miles 188 yards) is the most popular race distance in America, the ideal first race for all runners and joggers, and the logical goal for people not wishing to commit suicide due to inactivity. Do a gentle 2 to 3 miles per day on three days per week and running the 5K will be easy for you. It will also be an enjoyable way to extend your life, and you'll join 10 million other people who run more than 100 times per year.

A Harvard study showed that 24 minutes of intense aerobic activity gives you most of your cardiovascular fitness gains:

* You'll need to get into shape before you do those 24 minutes intensely.
* You'll need to warm up, stretch and cooldown after your 24 minutes of exercise.
* So, 40 minutes per "session" will keep you fit.

The goal of this book is to get you exercising regularly for about 40 minutes, and on some days, to have you do part of your session at moderate intensity. The goal is to exercise in comfort not pain.

A recent report from the Institute of Medicine in Washington D.C. recommends 60 minutes of exercise per day. They include yard work and cleaning your house as exercise, so don't stress your heart worrying about finding 60 minutes every day. However, do release the weekly maid service and gardener if you use them. When you reach 40 minutes of aerobic exercise on 5 days per week you'll be in the top 15 percent of the United States for fitness. Eventually, you can cruise up toward 60 minutes every day if you like...and rehire a gardener, but lets get you to the more modest 30 to 40 minute goal first.

Start slowly if you're overweight. Start just as slowly if you're not overweight! Start even slower if you have cardiac disease. You're 10 times less likely to suffer a cardiac event during exercise if you are healthy. If you have heart disease, start very slowly and only after medical clearance. Your risk will go down as you lose weight and get fitter.

Before reading beyond this page, put on a pair of shoes and walk for 2 to 3 minutes away from your chair <u>without</u> getting short of breath and without hurting. Walk back and do a few gentle stretches. Congratulations. You've found the time for an exercise program. Read on because your second session is in 48 hours.

Most best selling exercise books are written by celebrities or former couch potatoes who get it together for a year while selling a book, or make a career from endorsing exercise equipment.

Isn't it better to take advice from a lifetime exerciser rather than a new exerciser who probably will not be exercising next year when you are looking for inspiration?

I've motivated myself to exercise all my life, not just for the two years prior to the publication of this little book.

I will not apologize for never being overweight or out of shape:

However, I will give you the tools with which you can get into shape, or get into better shape! Some caveats:

* The American College of Sports Education recommend that men over 40, women over 50 and anyone with symptoms or risk factors for heart disease see a doctor before beginning a vigorous exercise program. However, you will not be exercising vigorously for many weeks. So:

* Set modest, achievable, sustainable goals for you, not for a person who is 40 pounds lighter, 10 years younger or already walking two miles most days.

* Hint: Aim for about three hours of exercise per week by the end of the third month. Yes, you can start that slowly to reduce your coronary risk factors.

* Which means: add only 15 minutes of exercise each week to your current exercise level.

* By the end of the first month you'll be exercising for an hour each week, but only for 10 to 20 minutes per day. By the end of month four, you'll be exercising 4 hours per week!

Not exercising at present?

You'll do only 15 minutes the first week and only 30 minutes the second week, yet by the end of the first month you will amass two and a half hours of exercise.

Infomercials love to sell exercise equipment with lines such as "you'll feel the difference in your fitness level in just 28 days."

You will still feel the difference in just 28 days with this program. Why? Because you will do two and one half hours more exercise in the next 28 days than you did in the last 28 days. Most of you will also decrease your calorie consumption by 200 to 500 calories per day, and eat a more balanced diet (see Appendix II). Net result: You're already losing weight and getting fitter.

See Chapter One to get fit without aches and pains and in one of this books many quirks, see Chapter Three for another way to start.

Do this exercise for you, for how much better you will feel afterwards. Be patient, enjoy every exercise session by moving slowly, without getting short of breath, for sustainable healthful exercise.

Make fitness fun and you'll exercise often enough to reap the benefits. Train with friends for humorous conversation or enjoy the elements and scenery. Make exercise a pleasurable experience by doing it at modest intensity but build up to decent duration. A few minutes of sex is fine for teenagers, but the real pleasure comes from extended sessions at modest intensity. Even more so with running. Maybe you *can* run half a mile in three minutes…and collapse on the grass, but it's more fun to run 4 miles in 30 minutes. If your limit is a fast quarter mile in two minutes followed by exhaustion, your fun or enjoyable run will probably 3 miles in 30 minutes. Pleasure and a "runners high" come from exercising at less than maximum intensity.

Some pre-book reading tips:

Set modest goals for this week and this month, while also looking forward to how you will feel next year, when you will have 52 weeks of exercise in the bank.

Enjoy the achievement of finishing your first mile OR your first 20 minute run, and do some of your exercise outside.

Do most exercise at 60 to 75 percent of your maximum heartrate…about 120 to 140 per minute for most of us. After a few weeks, do some exercise at modest tempo, taking your heartrate to 80 percent of your maximum for a minute at a time…145 to 160 for most people and include hills for stronger muscles.

Cross train every week & run a variety of routes and distances.

Wear running shoes always, and after the first few weeks, wear running shorts for your running.

Make plans to see a healthier you in the mirror, then exercise often enough to make it happen. Keep exercising after you've made it happen...you should not need to lose 10 pounds after every winter. People at the Arctic research facility exercise regularly. So can you.

Review your goals every month and keep them simple. *Getting fit* is a nice goal, but writing down that you will exercise 4 times this week for 10 minutes, and increase by 5 minutes per week until you've hit 30 minutes is more specific, and according to sport psychologists, more likely to get you exercising.

Make your children proud of you: Be a role model for them and others.

Run longer or faster...as part of a graduated training program for a race, and then race a 5K several times a year, but take a day off from exercise each week to do something which is special.

Train with other people sometimes, but train by yourself on some days. Both have their merit. Push yourself fairly hard for a few minutes on some days while working on running form.

But, do not hammer your workouts. Don't even workout. Instead of working out...exercise. (see page 194)

Be fairly consistent! Don't feel like running for 40 minutes? Slip out for a 20 minute run and stride out for 30 seconds about four times at the halfway point. Now that's a fun run.

Eat healthful foods without going to extremes. Drink low calorie liquids by the pint each day, not by counting how many glasses! 8 glasses per day is insufficient for regular exercisers.

Only 30 percent of women age 18-49 get their heartrate up to a moderate level for 20 minutes on three days per week. You'll burn more calories by including modest intensity exercise instead of staying at easy effort for all 40 minutes of your exercise. "But wait," as those TV commercials say, get used to 40 minute sessions before you include more intense exercise.

Train wisely by adapting any program in this book to meet your needs and abilities.

Please, no heavy breathing and no achy muscles in the first few months. Keep your exercise easy and let your body adapt.

David Holt
Santa Barbara, July 4th, 2004

Chapter One

It's Time To

GET MOVING

Later in this Chapter I'll show you how to save time and move up from 15 minutes per day of gentle exercise. But what if you can't walk or jog for 15 minutes? It probably shows your first training error, namely, that you are trying to walk or jog too fast. Don't worry. Overtraining is the most common mistake the first time that a person exercises after a break.

Next time you try to walk or jog, start slower and for a minimal amount of time. Although the following program is based on easy walking or jogging, aqua-aerobic classes, elliptical trainers or a bicycle are just as good for your initial exercise, especially if you are overweight. Whichever exercise you do, restrain yourself to easy effort for the stipulated time. Substitute the machines for jogging once or twice a week if it suits you, or do part of your exercise on machines at any stage of an exercise program. Chapters 16 and 17 give copious advice on cross training.

Wearing a decent pair of walking or running shoes, here is how to approach your first 28 days of exercise.

Week One:
On Monday, Wednesday and Friday walk or jog slowly for 5 minutes without getting short of breath. That's all folks. No special clothing required. Just make the time and get away from people for 5 minutes of continuous slow movement. Unless you are a truly morose person with no priorities or life, there is always enough time in a day for the important things. You just have to decide

which ones are important. Make your 5 minute walk a priority and you'll do it.

Week Two:
Celebrate your weekend with a 10 minute walk or jog, then do a gentle 7 minutes on Mon, Wed and Friday for a 31 minute total.

Week Three:
Your 13th or 14th day of your new life is the second weekend and calls for a 15 minute walk or jog or mixture of both. Your three midweek sessions increase to 10 minutes each.

Week Four:
Graduate to 15 minute walk/runs for all 4 sessions, but you will still not be getting short of breath because your goal is continuous movement at only 60 to 75 percent of your maximum heartrate.
Congratulations. You've set yourself up to succeed with regular exercise.

Prefer a table format?

Week	Sat	Mon	Wed	Fri	
One:	0	5	5	5	
Two	10	7	7	7	
Three	15	10	10	10	
Four	15	15	15	15	minutes of movement

Some of you will prefer to exercise both days at the weekend, plus Tuesday and Thursday. Use the combination which works for you, the combination which is most likely to succeed. Prone to Friday happy hour with colleagues or rushing out of town most weekends? Friday would be a poor choice for exercise unless you do it before work!

Aerobic exercise improves your circulation and the health of your heart and many other essential glands, while keeping you fit for life.

However: Gentle Exercise is the key to Regular Exercise. You need to avoid the aches and pains from starting an exercise program too strenuously.

o   If having more energy and feeling good don't appeal to you, relegate this book to the bookcase.
o   If being healthier or losing weight or toning up is not your goal, move to another book.
o   If belonging to a minority is not your idea of fun, click away.

However, you can become part of the 15 percent of the nation who exercise regularly using these simple steps.

Start your exercise gently.

Walk slowly; lift light weights; ride a bicycle leisurely: hardly work up a sweat at all. Don't even get out of breath. If you do work up a significant sweat, you're moving too fast or possibly wearing too much clothing for the conditions.

Most people who give up on an exercise program give up because they start too harshly…or don't start at all because they are afraid to fail. Get up off the sofa and throw this book away. Phew, throwing the book away prevented you from beginning an exercise program! Still holding onto 5K Fitness Run? Okay then.

Taking an ill prepared body through a strenuous workout predestines you to failure. Your aches and muscle pains after the workout, plus the discomfort during the training can put even the most resourceful people off of exercise for long periods. Use your mental resources to hold back. Short easy walks will prepare your skeleton and muscles for future exercise, while also getting you into the habit of finding time for exercise. Give your musculoskeletal system and cardiovascular system a chance to change at their pace.

The best exercise gurus eschewed the "no pain no gain" philosophy before the Internet and Internet books were invented. There are 24 hours to each day; your initial goal is a mere 15 minutes on four of those days. One hour per week out of the glorious 168 hours which man has invented (we could have set up a 50 hour day and a 10 day week). One of our current hours is less than one percent of the week. Use some imagination, or organization, and 60 minutes are easy to find.

Exercise programs fail due to lack of planning and unrealistic goals. Make your changes a few minutes per week and at modest intensity and your exercise program will require minimal effort. If all your exercise feels like work, it is being done too fast or against too much resistance.

Try these time finding ideas.

Join your employers wellness program for a yoga class or midday fitness walk. No program? Take one friend out for a 10 minute walk and you've started an informal program...provided you do it again two days later and again next week.

500,000 women die from heart disease per year in the United States. One of their reasons for failing to exercise regularly is that they are too busy caring for other people to take care of themselves, yet many put on make-up for over half an hour and watch children play entire soccer or baseball games.

Laying the foundation to your health with exercise will lay the foundation to your face! Take a brisk walk during the second to fourth innings of a baseball game. Only watch the second half of the soccer game. You can cook stir fry chicken, vegetables and rice in about half an hour if you're very organized. Or run for 23 minutes and microwave a 380 calorie Uncle Ben's rice bowl during your 7 minute shower. Less chance of overeating too.

Here's a variety of ways to get in your 15 minute session.

After dropping the children off at school, or before picking them up, drive to a quite spot such as a park on your typical route to work or school.

Walk slowly for seven minutes. Look around; take in the sights and sounds and smell that rose you've been ignoring for years, watch the ducks circle, or dogs running. After a one minute look, smell and rest, walk leisurely back to your car. Congratulations, you have just started your pain free exercise program.

Do something different: two days later, take your 15 minute walk at lunchtime. If you can find 3 to 4 flights of stairs to walk up also (do them slowly), you've just added strength training. Four flights of 15 steps at five inches per step means a 150 pound "weight lifter" has lifted 9,000 pounds!

The next day, leave work earlier than normal, or get home later to make space for your 15 minute stroll. Unwind as those work thoughts drift through your system. Use your work-stress adrenaline to send you 7 minutes to a viewpoint...then practice deep breathing as you force your work life out, and look toward your private time, to your healthful evening.

Two of the above sessions require that you keep exercise equipment in your car. Always have a set of exercise equipment in your car and a set at work. Shoes, shirt, socks, shorts and a towel are sufficient. You'll seldom have an excuse to miss exercise.

Your fourth session will be at the weekend. You only need to convert one half of one percent of your weekend into an exercise period. Do fifteen minutes out of your 48 hours with your heartrate up a few dozen beats per minute. You can break those fifteen minutes up if you wish. Research shows that you gain almost as much health benefit from exercising in short sections as you do from one continuous walk. You can park half a mile from the mall to give a total of a mile walk, or use the same trick for church. It might also discourage you from buying things you don't need because you'll have to carry them back to the car.

Talk is cheap, but exercise is also inexpensive. You only need to make a small time commitment to exercise regularly. Organize your life for a healthier life. Chapter 16 shows cheap ways to start weight training. Too cold to run outside? Indoor shopping malls cost you nothing if you move quickly and don't carry any money. A skipping or jump rope costs only a few dollars and builds up your calf muscles.

Increasing your aerobic exercise beyond 15 minutes per day. As you reap the benefits from this first hour of exercise every week, you'll begin to get fitter.

During the second month of regular exercise, you add 3 to 4 minutes per session each week, building to 30 minute sessions. In month three, you'll slowly increase to 40 minutes, 3 to 5 times per week. You'll begin to feel and look better, and also decrease your death risk from heart attacks, stroke and dozens of other ailments as shown in Appendix I, while increasing your overall health.

You can also increase intensity with somewhat faster walking or jogging in the middle 10 minutes of half of your sessions. When walking up those stairs, take them still slower, but two steps at a time. Stair walking will work your buttock muscles. After a few more weeks, add an extra flight or two, or take the elevator down then walk back up. You've just started interval training.

You only need to go up 11 flights of stairs Monday to Friday, to burn 100 calories per week, which is 1.5 pounds of fat every year and will give you a more muscular looking butt. Walk up but take the elevator down to save your back and your knees.

Then, add variety with gentle biking, swimming, skating (any kind you like), exercise machines or easy paced running.

You can add intensity by walking hills instead of stairs. However, don't take your heartrate above 80 percent of your maximum until you've been exercising for 3 months. Then, find a 2 to 5 percent incline and walk at your regular pace up the hill. Try shorter steps at first. If you use a treadmill, simply raise the incline gradually to about 6 %. Add another one percent every couple of weeks until your form vanishes, then go back one percent to your natural comfort zone. Do the middle third of your exercise session at this higher intensity. The majority of your exercise time should still be at 60 to 75 % of your maximum heartrate.

What is your maximum heartrate?

Somewhere between 220 and 200 beats per minute, depending on whether you were born 40 days ago or 40 years ago.

If you're not used to regular exercise, *maximum* exercise heartrate is usually based on 220 minus your age. Fit from years of training 5 hours per week? Your maximum is probably closer to 220 minus half of your age.

Unfit people train at a lower heartrate initially to avoid cardiac arrests, an unhealthy side effect of exercising too intensely when out of shape. It also decreases the risk of shin splints or shin pains, the number one injury of the new walker or runner.

Unfit and forty?

220 minus 40 = 180 (your maximum: stay away from here)
180 x 60 % = 108 (stay here in the early weeks)
180 x 80 % = 144 (don't reach this level for several weeks)
Stay mostly at the low end until you can exercise for at least 30 minutes. Be able to talk at all times as you ease your body toward fitness. The talk test is a very reliable predictor that you're at the right exercise intensity. After a few weeks you'll be walking or biking faster to reach that 108 to 144 pulse target.

Fitter people have to train at a higher heartrate to get a training affect. Fit people are also safer from the side effects of training more intensely. Their hearts are bigger and stronger, pumping out a huge volume of blood with every beat. For the most part, you are past the high risk point for cardiac arrests...unless you exercise too long, get dehydrated or ignore that persistent indigestion, family history of clogged arteries and fail to get an annual check up.

Formula for the fit people.

220 minus (half of 40) = 200

200 x 60 % = 120

200 x 80 % = 160

If being in shape to exercise safely at 140 beats per minutes for an hour at a time is punishment, you should take it! You can also factor in your heartrate at rest to get your "heartrate reserve".

Heartrate reserve (HRR) is: max HR – resting HR

Use the percentage of HRR + your resting HR for your target intensity. This competitive runner of three decades prefers the more simplistic percentage of maximum HR.

Think you can burn more calories by working at 90 percent of your maximum heartrate? You can...provided you still exercise for the same length of time. Lets say that you run four miles in 40 minutes with your heartrate at 140. Increase pace to 170 beats per minute for the middle 20 minutes, and to keep the arithmetic simple, you may be at 8 minutes per mile, giving you 4.5 miles for your session. That extra half a mile will burn about 50 calories. Hardly worth it you may think. Do this session twice a week for a year and your muscles will be stronger, plus you'll burn 5,200 calories, or about 1.5 pounds of fat. In ten years, you'll be 15 pounds lighter!

Your 170 heartrate section will probably be at or above anaerobic threshold, which as you'll see in Chapter 8 is one of the finest exercise intensities at which to train. Ease up to those twenty minutes over several sessions after starting with 5 minutes at the higher heartrate. Your ideal intensity may be 160 beats per minute. Aim for 85 to 90 percent of your maximum heartrate for these sessions, but don't do them every day.

A bonus to high intensity training is that your metabolism stays higher for longer than with gentle exercise. Thus, your calorie burn is still higher. There are two problems with training at higher intensities:

1. You need to get fit enough to train intensely. Doing excessive amounts of high intensity running, too early in your training leads to fatigue, burn-out and probably the end of your exercise program. You still need to do most of your exercise at modest intensities. You can't train at high intensities every day.

2. Some so called "Experts" say that you burn less fat with high intensity exercise. This is only true during the actual exercise...because the body uses mostly sugar during intense work bouts. However, you burn more calories (from sugar) during intense exercise. And where do you think the body is going to get new sugar from? Some of your well stored fat will be metabolized while you are walking round the supermarket, saving your sugar for your next workout. Your next carbohydrate meal will restock your glycogen store instead of being converted to fat.

If you're allergic to heartrate goals, use <u>Rate of Perceived Exertion</u> or RPE. No movement scores zero out of 20. Maximum effort scores 20. Laying on a sofa is a rest day; sprinting 100 meters to collapse is over exertion unless your event is less than 200 meters. The main area for runners is a score of 10 to 16 out of 20.

RPE	Effort level	Uses
10 to 11	Fairly light	Until you are fit enough to run for 30 minutes.
12 to 14	Somewhat hard	Wait until Chapter Five.
15 to 16	Hard	Chapter Seven and beyond.
17 and above.		After you've raced a couple of 5Ks or during Chapter 10 & 11.

A second RPI is based on a maximum score of 10. Thus:
*   1-2 is very easy, talking is not an effort.
*   3 requires minimal effort to talk.
*   4 is moderately easy. You need a little effort to converse. Don't go above this level until you can handle 30 minute runs.
*   5-6 is moderate to moderately hard, and talking will be in smaller sentences because it requires effort. You're probably at Chapter 7 or 8s level and over 80 percent of maximum heartrate. You should not be running here for several months.

* 7-8 is 5K racing or the sessions of Chapter 10 & 11 with talking a rare thing because you're exercising at a high intensity.
* 9-10 is for mile racers who are renowned for 2 word sentences when someone pushes them in a race. Stay away from here.

Most of your early running should feel easy. Don't get severely short of breath or end up with achy muscles the next day. You don't need to push your body to extremes to get fitter or faster:

o Fitter means fitter for life with greater endurance and strength and is best achieved with gentle runs at 60 to 70 percent of maximum heartrate, plus modest amounts of weight training with light weights.
o Faster means that you're able to run close to your maximum speed for a greater period of time. Most people can run at close to maximum speed for 50 meters to catch a bus. When you are fit enough to run faster, you'll be able to run at maximum speed for 200 meters, and close to maximum speed for an entire 5K.

Cruise through the next few chapters and gradually bring in quality exercise to burn more calories, but also add to the amount of time that you spend exercising. If you add ten minutes, five days per week to your current 4 miles in 40 minutes, you've got an extra five miles or 500 calories burned per week, for a yearly loss of about 7.5 pounds. Adding 10 minutes per day to your current zero or to your current 15 minutes per day of exercise will still burn 500 calories per week!

Having a purpose for your exercise and seeing yourself succeed will help you to "do it" often enough and for long enough to be useful. If you started with walking, you can convert to running slowly for one minute out of every five. After a couple of weeks, alternate 2 minute runs with 3 minute walks, and transition to 10 minute runs with one minute walks over the next three months.

Chapter Two

Excuses, Excuses

There is no acceptable excuse which prevents you from exercising.

It comes down to:

MOTIVATION

Believe that your running, walking or other exercise program will improve your physical state and your health...and it probably will. Be optimistic about your exercise program and it will be successful. It's up to you to overcome the occasional problem, and to keep moving forward a day at a time for a lifetime of fitness.

Running too far, too fast or too often results in injury and the loss of motivation to run.

There are minimal boundaries in running. You'll only discover your boundaries by gradually increasing mileage and then increasing your intensity. You have huge possibilities for improvements in fitness and health in the early days and years, and maintenance of health in later years of running.

Poor planning can make you dread each up coming run. Yet, if you stretch properly and regularly, increase your mileage and quality running in a logical and gentle way, all runners can maintain their motivation to run.

Beginners need a reason to start. Jumping into a marathon training program because 20,000 runners in a race inspired you to run a marathon is a bad idea. For the 85 percent of Americans who can't run three miles, a fun-run 5K also requires restraint.

Apart from wanting the fun and camaraderie from being with hundreds of like minded people, why spend time exercising?

* You'll live longer, with better eyesight, hearing and fewer disabilities. You'll sleep better, especially if you exercise outdoors, 2 or more hours before bed at moderate intensity.
* Improve your sex life as you become healthier and your feeling of self-worth improves. Circulation to your sex glands improves. People who exercise regularly are almost twice as likely to have sex in each week.
* Retain mental ability longer.
* You'll be more productive at work if you're physically fit. You'll take fewer sick days and be more satisfied at work.

See Appendix I for more detailed health benefits from exercise. Here are your tips on actually getting out for your exercise and staying with the program. The technical aspects mentioned in this chapter are explained later.

Make a date...to exercise.

You're more likely to continue with exercise if you enjoy it. The health benefits and calories burned are a bonus to the joy of exercise. Preparation plus the right attitude makes for achievement. Make regular exercise a habit, and you're more likely to stick with it. At 4 pm, you should not be thinking, "Shall I exercise this evening," because it sets you up for a refusal. Instead, think, "What exercise shall I do today." If you set say, Monday, Wednesday and Friday as your 45 minute exercise sessions, you only have to decide whether to run, walk or do 25 minutes of weight training followed by biking or elliptical training on these days. While you should do something else special for yourself on the three exercising days, Tuesday and Thursday could be your non-exercising special treats such as a movie or cooking that special meal...of 10 servings to give you healthful entrées for your freezer.

No time to exercise?

It's your life, so it's up to you how you use each of those 36 segments of 40 minutes per day. Make exercise a priority.

* Get up 40 minutes earlier;

* Organize your lunch hour better;
* Bicycle to work and back twice a week;
* Pick up the children half an hour later from child care;
* Force your child to do his or her own homework;
* Let your significant other do dinner. You can exercise indoors while monitoring the last three! Or go for a 30 minute run.

The options are endless. Running is more likely to happen if you write down your training time-block and don't let other, less important activities intervene. Exercise is vital, so do it.

Tricks to finding time for healthful exercise.

Write down what you watch and for how long you watch TV. Figure out why you watch TV and then donate all but one of your TVs to a charity! Decide on the best time to switch on your remaining TV.

Record how much work you do at home. An employer has no right to your lunchtime or your free time. They are not entitled to an explanation as to why you cannot do a task which is so important to them...right now. You do not have to give an excuse for being out at lunch time, or for leaving at 5 p.m. if that is your scheduled finish time. People working the essential services do have rules to guide them, but most workers can leave the work place on time.

Exercise while your children are doing their sport. You'll be back in time to cheer them on during the rest of the game.

Or, take the children with you on your walks. Listen to the highlights of their day while starting them on an exercise program. Children who exercise, just like adults who exercise, are less likely to do drugs...both the illegal and the legal drugs tobacco and alcohol (which kill ten times as many people as the illegal drugs).

Prepare the lunchtime food before bedtime; set out the breakfast things; decide on tomorrows clothing and place it ready to put on; set your alarm 22 minutes early so that you can make whoopee. OOPS, I mean to go walking or running prior to breakfast. Set limits on other people using your time.

There is stacks of time at the weekend...provided you make exercise as big a priority as the 8 to 10 meals you will be eating. Nobody needs to go to the mall, unless it is carpeted and open for exercise before the stores open on cold or hot days.

Feeling too tired to run? So what, go running anyway to get invigorated for the rest of your day and the rest of your life.

A study of women who exercised with brisk walking released in August 1999, showed a magnificent decrease in heart attacks. To get the full health gains from exercise, you will eventually need to work up a light sweat for 20-30 minutes. Increase intensity slowly, by a few minutes per week and you can keep your exercise a pleasurable experience.

Get away from the Internet.

You do not have to check e-mail every hour let alone every 10 minutes. Check it twice a day if you must. If it's urgent, the person can telephone you...can't they. Talk in person to save typing time. Don't waste time opening most of the e-mails. Peruse the sender addresses and subject matter and move the ones you're going to read to a reading file. Select "edit all" and "delete" to get rid of the rest in one go.

Looking something up on the Internet? Use an appropriate phrase in a quality search engine and peruse the sample paragraph or titles before choosing one or two sites to check. Get off the Internet after 10 minutes if you have not found decent information.

Save time by training on your own.

It can take 30 minutes longer to do a 6-mile run with friends. Commutes and waiting for the second or third person, different stretching and warm up exercise wants, and the discussion about the running route can burn the clock!

But do run with other people sometimes.

The commitment to run with them helps you to keep your date to run. Stretch and warm up while waiting. Add some relaxation and deep breathing exercises. Start at the designated time and run the same mile at the start each week so that late comers know where you've gone and can meet you on the way back. They can also park at the one mile point and join in.

Speed running feels easier with company. One famous running quote is that killer track sessions are easier in a group.

However, even experienced runners should not be running killer track sessions. You need gentle sessions at 5K pace, (see

Chapter Eleven) not kill the runner, and make no improvement to your 5K racing potential sessions at mile race pace. Instead of running flat out, run at appropriate pace for you, especially when training with other runners.

Most running should be slow enough to allow you to talk. If the running doesn't keep you out of therapy, chatting and laughing with friends should.

On some days, run with someone who is slower than you are. Run at their pace, but don't let them race. On another day, run with someone who is a bit faster than you are. Again, no racing, but this may be your day at tempo pace.

Extroverts should run on their own sometimes to enjoy a little solitude and actual thinking instead of mixing with other people. Introverts should join a running club and seek out fellow runners for company. You all enjoy running, so this is a great chance to talk, listen and mix with other people while feeling comfortable.

Increasing your Training?

Managing OK with 5-mile runs? Mileage is the biggest predictor of injury, so add some gentle speed running at 5K race pace. Speed running at modest paces teaches your body to run properly and efficiently, which decreases injury risk. Been running regularly for several months? Done several 5K races? Increase your endurance by edging up to 10 miles once a week.

Find running 10 miles easy? Race some 10Ks and consider higher mileage programs such as the ones shown in *10K & 5K Running, Training & Racing.*

No enthusiasm for long runs?

Don't do them! Fifty to 60 minutes runs, twice a week is sufficient to enjoy 5K fun-runs. Do a little cross training and weight training and you'll be ahead of 90 percent of the population. However, don't race a 10K. Run a 10K conservatively for pleasure or it will hurt too much. Race at the 5K.

You'll get slightly more health benefits from running 30 miles per week if you include a run of 10 miles.

Want to run 10 miles? Enjoy the party by:

* Adding half a mile to your longest run every other week.
* Run interesting routes for scenery, sounds and activity.

* Run part of it with a friend...at appropriate pace for you.
* Think about your running form each mile, especially the last few miles, but think and talk about other things too.
* Start very slowly. Run the first mile a minute slower than your average pace, then ease up to 60 to 75 percent of your maximum heartrate.
* Wander through woods, paths and somewhat familiar areas to ramble. However, carry liquid and energy and know where you are in that last half an hour. You need to reach your car or bus stop at about 10 miles, not 13.
* Use positive feedback and self-talk to get through long runs. Telling yourself you can do something becomes a self-fulfilling prophecy...especially if you stay hydrated, and only run one mile farther than your longest run of the last month. Or you run the same distance, but only five seconds per mile faster than last month.
* Long runs are a chance to daydream about your running form, your capabilities at the 5K, and to solve that nagging problem...the answer can jump into your mind at any point: pure inspiration creates your solution. At a minimum, you'll get a significant break from your emotional problems.
* Take a bus or train out 10 miles, and run back. Generally, you should have cut-offs available. You should be able to turn a 10 mile run into a seven if things go wrong.

Don't feel guilty about using your cut-offs. You need to avoid exhaustion. You'll also be fresher for quality running over the next few days. You can judge the right speed for you on the next long run. Don't try to catch up on this missed long run if you're preparing for a 10K. The 8th run at 10 miles over a 14 week period would help...a bit. Sometimes, one less long run is better.

While getting ready for a 10K race, continue to have fun with 5Ks once a month. Remember to take a day off weekly to do something special for yourself.

Don't feel guilty about the time you spend running. It makes you a better person for the rest of the day.

Don't get greedy.

After races, take at least a day off from fast running for every kilometer that you raced. Enjoy restive runs at 70 % of max HR.

Always getting injured?

You've probably increased mileage or speed too rapidly. Cross train gently at 70 percent of max HR: don't take out your frustration on an elliptical machine by training at 90 % of your max HR the first week; find the cause of your injury, do the rehab exercises recommended and be patient because you will run again.

Have several goals.

Your main goal can be the big 5K race, which takes place in conjunction with the cities marathon in nine months. The goal which gets you out the door will need to be a smaller 5K race in 2 to 3 weeks, or the 5 mile run with friends most Sunday mornings, or a quick three mile run on Tuesdays, or doing enough running to keep you in shape to do any of the previous three.

Your goals must be realistic.

Running 28 minutes for 5K after your first six months training? 27 minutes is a realistic goal in another six months. Running 28 minutes after 5 years of training? You'll need to look closely at your training to find out if something is missing. Then make the changes gradually to be able to run faster. Staying under 28 minutes could be your goal. However, running 5 seconds per mile faster may be an option. To improve you'll probably need to leave the comfort zone by running some miles a bit faster. You'll probably need to reduce the recovery when doing Interval training. See Chapters 5 to 11.

Run at the best time of day for you.

I have a physical job, nursing. I usually work two 12 hour shifts per week. These are my days off from running, though I may do 30 minutes of elliptical training on one work day. The other 5 days are for running and writing. On two of the 5 days I also cross-train.

Keep a weekly training log for inspiration.

Include the time at which you ran, the weather (if unusual), running pace, companions and place of running or route. You can include much more, but don't make it a chore.

As you age you will eventually slow down.

As your performances drop in terms of speed, your training pace should decrease too. But whatever age you are, you can still train at this years 5K pace and this years 15K pace (15K or 10 mile race is 30 to 40 seconds per mile slower than 5K pace).

Don't race all the people in each race.

You can ignore racing most runners in your age group, or only race against those in your age group. Age 42? Race against the 42 and older athletes...but take care, many of them are very experienced. Note: You'll also be surrounded by younger runners but you don't need to race them. You can use each other to have a great race.

The 40s to 70s are the best decades of your life. You have experience and some of you are sensible about your training!

There are great athletes in all 5-year age groups. You can compete against some of them, or against a realistic time target. It does not matter if you are in the top 10 percent in a race, or sneak into the top 90 percent. The training must be (mostly) enjoyable by being at the right intensity for you. While it's good to do some high intensity stuff to help your racing, do something on a daily basis which is physically undemanding for yourself also.

Run for stress relief.

Moving house or coping with bereavement? Run for relaxation and pleasure while using a simple exercise that reduces stress levels. Manage your life stress by dealing with them too. Don't let running add to your stress. Run fewer miles or less intensely when major events happen in your life. Ten weeks at 70 percent of your usual mileage, and running fartlek sessions in the woods or striders on grass instead of track sessions is a rest phase. You can still run with friends and do a 5K race one weekend a month for the social aspect of running. Make sure that your running partner will run slowly enough to keep your runs stress free. Stressed or not, run the first mile of all runs slowly. Run the first mile of all races five seconds slower than your expected average pace for that distance.

Note: A 4-mile tempo run may be what you desire with your friend. Make sure it is the right tempo for you. Retain a small amount of fast running at 5K pace each week and you'll lose less fitness than with only slow miles.

Run when you're on vacation.

You have the time. There's usually something you don't want or need to do with your family. You have different places to see and experience, so see some of them on foot. Take one new pair of running shoes to break in and they'll be ideal for speedwork on the third run and a long run a few days later; take an old pair for short runs. Take along some dead tee-shirts and your oldest socks to trash after your runs, and your suitcase will be lighter and odor free for your return home.

Vacations are an opportunity to engross your exercise...you don't have those 40 to 60 hour work weeks to distract you. Plan for running to be a natural part of the vacation experience. Running is an excellent way to view a new area. It will do you and the family good to manage without you for an hour a day.

If you believe exercise is the healthiest thing you can do for yourself, then you should still run or cross train five days a week while away from home. Check a map first and see some of the sights or head to the parks or trail heads. Slip in some fartlek, long reps, or 20 minutes of tempo running if the terrain asks you to.

Run in fun places when not on vacation.

This is your 40 to 60 plus minutes to be yourself. Trails encourage modest paced running: Find trails with soft surfaces to reduce the impact from whacking your body back onto the planets surface hundreds of times per mile. Run with a light step upon the surface. Despite the fact that your effort level will be the same...60 to 75 percent of your maximum heartrate, you'll be running a little slower, and your injury risk is lower. To remain ready for road races, do a small proportion of running on the road at close to race speed to practice pace judgment and running form.

Unusable Excuses to stay on the sofa:

I'm too old to exercise: Start regular exercise at any age and you'll improve muscle strength and overall fitness for life. Within weeks, you'll also decrease your death risk from numerous diseases. You will feel younger. You can turn your aerobic fitness clock back 30 years or more. You can even compare your 5K times at any age with what you could have done as a younger person.

Age graded tables are available via www.runnersworld.com or
www.runningtimes.com

It will take you 5 years to reach your best physical 5Ks if you
start exercise after age 40, then you can maintain the same age
graded standard for the rest of your life.

I'm overweight: 64.5 percent of the U.S. is overweight; leave
their well padded behinds, behind by walking short distances. Add
distance and increase pace gradually. Walk on sand to increase the
calorie burn by 60 percent, but decrease speed for your early sand
sessions to avoid overtraining.

Exercise does burn calories, but weight loss is determined by
consuming fewer calories than you burn for the entire month.
Enjoy your treats, but take them in moderation, or as a reward for
achievements in your running such as:

* 5 runs this week, or
* Achieving 15 miles in back to back weeks, or
* Running two times one mile at 85 to 90 percent of your
  maximum heartrate for the first time.

Running hurts too much: Pain means you're running too
fast. Warm up for ten minutes with a short walk and ease into slow
running while singing a song. Singing or talking will discourage
you from running faster than conversation pace. Can't talk because
you are moving too fast? Stop running and walk a few hundred
yards. Start running again but slower. Until you can run five miles
without aching the next day, add no more than a couple of minutes
or a quarter of a mile to the length of your longest run in a week.
When you are ready to move beyond 5 miles, add another half mile
every other week.

You will often have slight aches from a prior days solid yet not
too demanding session. Engross the slight soreness, which is the
result of a sensible increase in training volume or intensity, but be
careful to what degree you ache.

Muscles giving you pain signals? Don't take analgesics before
runs to shut off the pain. Ease the pace, ice and read the injury
advice in *Running Dialogue* or *Best Marathons*. Use an ice pack or
frozen peas for 10 minutes at a time or use a cold wrap from
www.liquidice.biz

Start your exercise program gently. No hurting people. You'll be exercising again tomorrow!

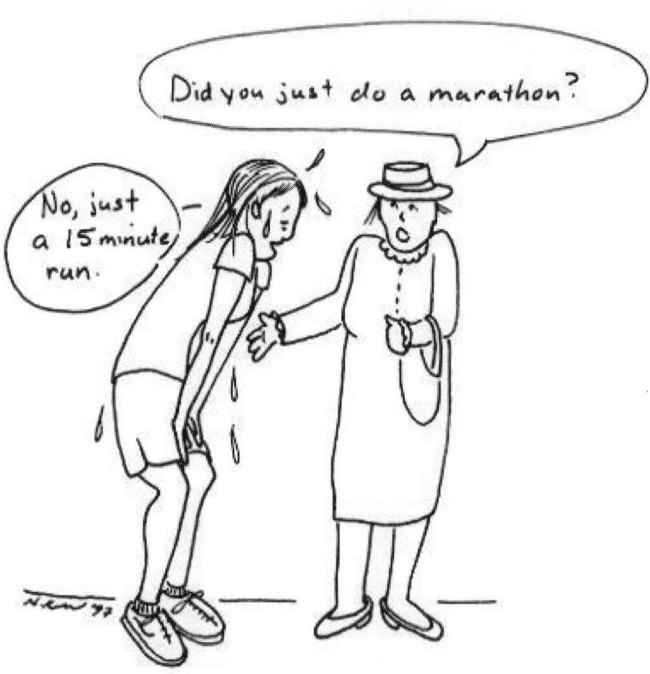

<u>Too cold to run:</u> Start with a thin layer of breathable synthetic material such as CoolMax, which wicks perspiration away from your skin. Use several layers, and top them off with a windproof exercise jacket. Cover your legs too. You're over dressed if you sweat a huge amount when training. Wear mittens for finger comfort.

During cold spells, arrange to meet a friend for some runs. Warm-up indoors, then put your winter garb on and head out to lighted streets, malls or sports arenas and college tracks. Alternatively, run short loops from your house or work place if the weather has a tendency to sudden changes. Reward yourselves with cocoa made with non-fat milk and plan for that warm climate vacation spot or your summer runs.

Nastiest winter in the Northeast or Rockies in 80 years? Stop complaining and get on with some cross training with snow shoes or cross country skiing and other Chapter 17 options such as treadmill running.

Too hot to run: It can be over 20 degrees cooler 10 miles away if there is a body of water, or mountains, or woods or other shaded areas away from concrete and asphalt. A forest can be worth an SPF-10 sunblock. Stripe down to the minimum, carry water, and run slower. Don't wear cotton. Gyms usually keep their training areas below 80 degrees and many are as low as 60.

Stay hydrated. You are more likely to consume liquid if it's cool and has a nice taste. However, warm liquid is absorbed just as quickly according to recent studies, so warm liquids will be fine if they keep you rolling. You don't have to buy sports drinks. Dilute 12 ounces of your favorite fruit juice with 20 ounces of water and you'll get the 200 calories which a quart of sports drink provides. The juice will provide more nutrients too. Avoid fruit juice blends and cocktails because they contain very little fruit juice and lots of fructose; same for sports drinks with fructose which can upset the stomach. If you're used to caffeine, it will not dehydrate you. Coffee before training is not a problem, but take a water chaser on hot days and see page 221.

Or run in water: Water reduces injury risk from ground impact and you stay cool (pages 169-172). Or use a treadmill or elliptical trainer in a room that is cool enough and has a fan (pages 174-178). Bicycle riding sets up a greater cooling effect than running, plus you can carry more liquid (pages 178-183).

Too lethargic: Exercise is invigorating, and the energy boost lasts longer than the boost from a candy bar. A steady run gives you more energy to cope with life and is an anti-depressant. You'll feel better about yourself and gain confidence after running. It takes strength of character to overcome inertia and take the first step out of the door.

Winter getting you down? Do some of your runs in daylight to increase your brain's serotonin levels, and beat the winter blues. The guy who was 15 seconds ahead of you in those 5K races last fall may not be out running this month; you will be out, and you'll run faster in the spring because you maintained fitness throughout the winter. You won't have to struggle to regain fitness or to lose excess weight in the spring if you keep running and cross training in the winter. Running, just like breathing, is a year round sport.

Too busy to run: So what, so am I. Lace on your training shoes and you can walk or run from your door. You need no other equipment or a commute to the gym. You shower once or twice a day anyway, so exercise for 30 minutes before you shower. Too busy means that you are too disorganized!

Too busy...two: Taking up a new activity will force you to be more organized, or you will decrease the time you spend doing something you don't need to do. You learn to prioritize. Want to strengthen your mind, body and live longer...then get off your gluteal muscles and walk or bicycle or run on a regular basis.

Start with ten minutes of walking a day. Ten minutes will make a difference and soon turn into 20 minutes or more. While 20 minutes will give you many of the health benefits from exercise, 30 minutes is where the real fun begins. A subtle exercise high creeps into your body because your endorphin and anandamide levels rise; the latter gives you a buzz while also dilating your bronchioles and arteries to make your running feel easier.

I have no friends who run: Running is your friend. Running is always there and is even more dependable than a dog. However, go to a track, and to several 5K races, and you'll soon find some running friends.

No one runs at my speed: A person who runs a 17 minute 5K can run with Olympic runners and with 10 minute per mile runners...for part of their runs. Potential running partner faster than you? No problem. Find out when his or her easy day is. Run with them on that day, but let them do the talking...because you will be running hard to keep up. Don't race them. Run even pace about half a step behind so they know who is setting the tempo. Your running goal can be different, yet you're still compatible for one or two runs per week. You can also join a running club and find people closer to your level. The Road Runner's Club of America is at www.rrca.org

I'm intimidated by faster runners: Someone has to be the slowest. Once you've done a couple of Interval sessions from Chapter 11 on your own, join a running group at the track. Don't run so fast that you hurt in the early sessions. Don't run more than 5 seconds per mile faster than your usual speedwork in the early sessions. The only person you need to impress is yourself. Other runners will only be impressed if you run:

* Most of your repeats at an even pace;
* Your last repeats at the same speed as your first repeats;
* Without pushing or barging through the group.

It's your race times, not your interval times which impress others.

When the fast guys and dolls are training at their 5K pace, you can train at your 2-mile effort. Or when they run half miles, you can run quarters at the same speed and get a huge rest period. During mile repeats you can also take a 10 second start and run two laps at your 5K pace while they catch you up at their 5K pace, then you can finish with one lap at their speed, or your 2-mile pace. This is called a differential. It teaches your muscle fibers to be efficient when you are tired. You can then walk as you watch them run their 4th lap at speed. In six months, you may be ready to run 600 meters at their speed.

If a group is big enough, it will split into several training levels. This author has been the slowest in the pack while training for 53 minute 10 mile races and 15 minute 5K racing. This author has been one of the fastest in a group while training for a 62 minute 10 miles and 18 minute 5Ks.

Running is boring: Breathing is boring, but we do it almost every minute. Find new running routes and notice different things on each run. Stop for a stretch and enjoy the view. Run close to nature, and run as close to natural as the elements allow.

Track or speed sessions are boring: Never repeat a speed session until three weeks after you last did it. Never repeat a speed session until three weeks after you last did it. That's not an editing mistake. Twelve times 400 meters at 5K pace is an excellent session, but the next week you should run something along the lines of 15 x 300 meters at 2 mile pace (10 to 16 seconds per mile faster than the 400s). The third week could be 6 x 600 meters at 5K pace, followed by 8 relaxed 200s just a bit faster than 2 mile pace (no more than 8 seconds per mile faster).

Do a fartlek session on grass with 45 to 90 second efforts at 5K pace the fourth week and you'll be ready to repeat the track sessions. Do a mixture with your long repeats too: Repeats of 2 miles at 15K pace, 2,000 meters at 10K pace, 1,000 meters at 5K pace give variety while stimulating all of your energy systems.

It's too early to run: Not every person wants to run within fifteen minutes of waking up. Placing your running shoes by your bed, plus sufficient other gear to stay warm enough on the run makes the choice a commitment rather than a choice.

Setting your coffee maker to wake you up can help. Dilute the coffee with non-fat milk to give yourself a few calories. Place a glass of water at the bedside and you can do more rehydration before you stumble toward the bathroom. Limbering up and stretching should wake you up enough to be safe in that crucial first 400 meters. This is the most familiar 400 meters and the most likely time for you to forget to look for traffic.

Early runs can be invigorating, but dress for the conditions. It should take monstrous rains or frozen water to keep you inside. If conditions are atrocious, use the time to do something you would have been doing later. You'll free up that later time for exercise.

Too late to run: Stop procrastinating and "do it." Late runs are cooler in summer. You'll need more clothing and reflective gear plus a flashlight in winter. You can run two hours after a light meal, but run with safety in mind. Be seen, run in the safest areas with little traffic, and face on-coming vehicles. Many running tracks are lit in winter. Indoor training works too of course.

Too tired from yesterdays run: You're supposed to be tired after some runs. Walking benefits runners...so walk half a mile. Running at 60 percent of maximum heartrate is better than walking...so run easy for two to five miles, then walk to finish. However, do take a day off once a week.

Speedwork feels like work: Don't feel like doing a track session? That's okay, read the Fartlek section in Chapter Five. You can do your fast running almost anywhere. Of course, you may simply need to run slower at the track! If you know the purpose of the session and run the first few repeats at the right pace, your positive self-talk will see you through the rest of the session.

My significant other does not like me to exercise:

Provided you're a non-smoker, regular exercise is the best thing you can do to preserve a healthy life.

If a one hour break from your partner twice a week, and a 40 minute break three days a week pull you away from your partner, consider taking your 4 hours of exercise, plus the rest of your life away. Most people work 5 to 8 times longer than they workout. Guide and support your significant other toward their hobby.

You should overtly do some of your training to maximize quality time with your friends. The pre-breakfast or lunchtime easy run can free up your evening. You can also fit in a quality speed session in 40 minutes. Or get to your training spot earlier than normal, do your full session while avoiding the time wasting items, and get to your designated date spot in a timely manner.

I'm not getting any faster. Run primarily for the pleasure
of a particular run, not to get faster at an arbitrary race distance like the 5K. Be prepared for personal records to stagnate as your body adjusts to its training. Running is a process. Take the long view, and start a progressive training program specific to your needs.

Add some gentle speed running or take shorter rest periods during your current speedy sections for greater stimulation.

Medalists in August get there because of the background strength and endurance training the previous winter...and the prior ten years or more of training. A new runner can easily take 12 seconds off a 5K time with a 12 week training program. It takes more than a 12-week program to achieve great races.

It really is time for a rest? You need rest every week.
Most people get two days off from work. Unless you are taking running really seriously, apply the same rules to your sport. You can easily run 30 miles a week in five runs. Do a ten once and it leaves you five miles for the other four days. Two of the fives should include some gentle speed running, but don't make it speedwork; also, run against resistance such as hills or sand.

Take a 25 percent mileage drop one week in four to stay fresh and motivated. Take an easy month once a year while you learn to ski, or trail walk or take a biking vacation. Run moderately fast for three miles once or twice a week that month and you'll retain 75 percent of your running fitness. If your different activity is physical, prepare for them with specific exercises.

Enter a 5K race. Place the race details on your refrigerator or a less cluttered but frequently observed spot. It may decrease your ice cream binges too, though it's less effective than not buying ice cream in the first place! Tell people you are running the 5K in 2 months, and then you will have to do some training for it.

Be time efficient with speed running:
Most of this books speed sessions have you run 10 percent of your weekly mileage in one session, giving you up to 5 miles or up to 60 minutes with a warmup and cooldown. Do five minutes of easy running, then gradually increase pace toward 15K speed for 2 to 3 minutes a few times. After 20 minutes you'll be warmed up, so put in a few surges of 2 minutes at 5K pace, then cooldown.

My dog doesn't want to go running:
Yeah right! There will come a stage when your mutt slows down enough to stay with you for the entire run, instead of doing twice the mileage that you do. Until then, it will wag its tail at the mere hint of a run. There will come a time when he or she needs a walk instead of a run. It will then be time for another dog to keep the old guy company during its last days, and to run with you.

Putting Efficiency into Practice
High mileage AND low mileage runners need organization. Training schedules can be a major chore if the person has to pick up progeny from daycare within 10 minutes of regular work finish time. Yet, this may only need adjusting one day a week.

Monday can be the most fun. Whereas colleagues may have a miserable Monday back at work, the runner gleams because he or she spends the morning looking forward to a lunchtime run.

Thirty minutes of the hour are spent running, 15 in the park which is half a mile from work. On return to the building, the small towel and favorite brand of periwash or skin cleanser from the supermarket, or deodorant soap make rapid work of the perspiration. Though it'll be another 12 hours before bacteria would give even a hint of body odor, a little deodorant is applied.

The most likely person to claim you have body odor that afternoon is the moron who is jealous that you exercise at all, let alone that you're organized to do so in your lunch break.

You'll eat a healthful sandwich or low fat energy bar plus a piece of fruit in the remaining 15 minutes of the break, and be the sweetest smelling person in the afternoon conference. The only aura coming from this person is the satisfied post-run aura.

Tuesday evening...leave work early, or arrange to pick up the children later. Do your run in an area on the way home, even if it requires a short detour. If you're leaving work at 5 pm consider an energy bar, plus liquid at 3.30 pm to avoid that empty feeling just before you run. Breakfast and lunch would have fuelled your run, but a carb and protein afternoon snack makes you more likely to actually run at 5.30.

Thursday...it's pre-work exercise. This should help you through what many workers think is the most difficult day of the week. If the early rising knocks you out, find a quiet spot for half of your lunch-break, and take a healthy power nap. Doing your commute earlier may save you 50 percent of the time for an exercise session.

Doing all three runs at the same time of day may suit you. Be adaptable. Running home from the carpool site works for some. Getting dropped off five miles from the Sunday brunch spot can give the other spouse quality time with his or her parents. Dare to be different. Adapt to each problem.

Don't live vicariously. If explained to appropriately, a child will understand why you are running for half of the baseball game instead of putting on weight sitting in the bleachers. He or she may still pout and cry, but they are doing their sport for themselves, aren't they? They are not doing it for you. On the other hand, you *are* doing your exercise for them; regular exercise increases the chances of you seeing them graduate from college. Encourage their exercise with self exercise.

<u>Eat breakfast every day</u>: Breakfast sets you up for healthful eating the rest of the day. You'll say no to those 10 am donuts; you'll be alert all morning; you'll decline the high calorie pizza and eat healthfully at lunch.

But, the breakfast should be good for you. See the tips in Appendix II and stick with whole-wheat products, plus low-fat dairy, whole fruit and a few nuts.

As we have the space, here are a few more tips before you reach page 222.

* Weight train twice a week to build muscles which burns 50 calories every day for every extra pound.
* Share a meal when eating out or get a doggy bag when you order and put half of it away before you start eating.
* Eat slowly when out and at home because the message that you've had sufficient takes 20 minutes. Don't keep eating until you're full; stop when you're satisfied; don't empty your plate.
* Measuring cups. Learn portion size and portion control.
* Tomatoes, artichokes, broccoli, cauliflower, spinach, carrots, zucchini, green beans have very few calories for their volume. Eat these more often than peas, beans, and corn.
* Make friends with the grill; throw out the frying pan.
* Take a short walk instead of munching on processed foods.
* Don't have high calorie, processed or junk food in the house.
* Accept that you will have bad eating days. Start afresh the next morning with an orange and a large bowel of high fiber cereals.
* Slow down and be able to exercise for longer and burn more calories. Add 10 minutes of walking to your runs.
* Don't diet.

Chapter Three

THE EARLY RUNS

As you saw in Chapter One and Two, exercise is based on the overload principle.

* You exercise gently to a minimal level of fatigue;
* After a recovery phase of 30 hours to two days, exercise again.
* You gradually increase the amount of exercise which you do, or the resistance which you use.
* With appropriate rest, your muscles, skeleton and circulatory system will adapt.
* You're following Oregon's former coach Bill Bowerman's classic Hard/Easy approach to running.

As you can see on page 28, the first cartoon in this author's book *Running Dialogue* has an observant person asking a collapsing, heaving runner if she has run a marathon. The runner responds with, "No, I just ran for 15 minutes." The moral is to start regular exercise gently.

Able to walk 3 to 4 miles in an hour without a cardiac arrest, perhaps by using this authors *5K Fitness Walk,* or Chapter One of this book, you may be ready to run. During the first few weeks or months training, you will progress to run for 40 minutes, without stopping, several times a week. Those of you who can run for 40 minutes already can stride effortlessly to Chapter Five.

To be successful with an exercise program you must tell yourself that you can do it. Eighty-five percent of the nation cannot run 3 miles, so you're about to join an elite group. Fill your mind with images of jogging, running or walking effortlessly, then, provided you exercise at 60 to 70 percent of your maximum heartrate, it will usually be effortless while you exercise.

Positive images make for positive experiences. Think you're strong and powerful and you will be able to run two minutes longer than you did last week, and reach 40 minutes per run in a few months. Visualize efficient runners to run with better form.

Watch a large 5K race and you'll see all body types. Whether you walk the first mile, then run 500 meters of a 5K race and walk the rest, or run the entire 5K, you all get the sense of achievement from completing a race. You'll also get the same wonderful sense of achievement after every 3 to 4 mile walk or run.

Take control of your life with a few minutes of regular exercise to get the health benefits out-lined in Appendix I. Think about good running form as you ease your way through runs at easy effort. As your conditioning improves you'll be able to run farther or faster as detailed in the next few chapters.

There is nothing wrong with walking. Walking brings the same relaxation and health maintenance benefits as running. However, this is the running a 5K book, so you'll need to alternate running with walking in whatever ratio you like such as 5 minutes of each, or two minutes of walking for every 8 of running and eventually continuous running.

Walking is great preparation for running. Your muscles, from your brain which you use to get out of the door to your heart and calves will be in pretty good shape. All you need to do is run easily for a minute...then walk a minute...and alternate running and walking for the middle part of your loop.

As you get used to running, do two minutes run, one walk. With practice, you'll find the pace at which you can run easily. Increase the running part each week until the only walking sections are where you have a good view to enjoy.

As mentioned in the introduction, if you have any doubts about your health, go to see a doctor before your first exercise session. A 20 minute run is not the way to begin a fitness program if its been preceded by years of smoking, or drinking or eating to excess.

Exercising, rather than diet alone is the best way to lose excess weight. Those people who exercise while losing weight will maintain muscle mass better than those who lose weight with diet only. In addition, the low intensity exercise gets you started on your way to fitness while speeding your weight loss. Don't use exercise simply to lose weight. Exercise for fun, because it makes weight control easier, and contributes to your health. You may need to consume a bit more protein in your first 8 weeks of regular exercise. Your muscles are going to tone up or grow and you will make more red blood cells and blood volume. 2 grams per inch of height is sufficient, and you're probably already getting it.

A few weeks of walking, swimming and riding a bicycle, combined with weight loss if necessary and a cessation of smoking, should prepare your body for its first run.

Actually, you don't *have* to lose weight. Overweight people get the same health benefits from exercise that appropriate weight for height people get. Of course, it's tougher to run when you're carrying 20 or 200 pounds too much. Your HDL cholesterol and your heart will still improve, and you'll be fitter for life...compared to overweight non-exercisers.

If you're 5 feet tall and weigh 343 pounds you'll probably need a period of walking, cycling or elliptical training at low intensity to get your muscles into shape for exercising at 60 percent of your maximum heartrate, let alone running. Losing some of your excess weight will probably be needed before you run.

Set yourself short-term goals. For example:
Lose 10 pounds while walking a mile three times a week.
Reward yourself by adding a swim or two.
Lose another five pounds and the reward can be a bicycle...
Which lets you add two rides a week to lose more weight:
When your reward could be walking scenic, hilly trails.

Don't be too concerned with how you look when exercising because no one else is. Wear any old clothing initially.

If you get short of breath, or have chest pains while walking, seek a medical opinion before proceeding. Once you can walk 40 minutes without feeling tired, try running.

The first run should be at a gentle pace. Your breathing rate will go up a bit: please, no gasping for air.

Choose an area without hills and work out a route that takes half an hour to walk. Start running very slowly, and with short steps. If your breathing becomes labored...stop. Walk until your breathing is back to normal, then run slower. It may take many attempts before you find a pace that your heart and lungs can handle.

At this stage, all running should be at a pace which enables you to talk. If you cannot talk with reasonable ease, you're running too fast. Get around in comfort and create the hunger for more.

In addition to avoiding heart attacks and loss of interest due to starting out with too fast a run, you must avoid over-training. Runners often suffer from overtraining, which is usually due to too much mileage or training too fast.

* If you ran too fast in your first run?
* If you have aching muscles for days afterwards?
* You're having your first experience with over-training.

Pace yourself to enjoy the sensation of running without feeling exhausted during or after the run.

Stretching: To decrease slight aches from properly exercised muscles, stretch before and after running. This maintains your flexibility, allowing a full range of movement, and reduces injury risk. Some people prefer to say that your muscles and tendons are more elastic, or possess elasticity with regular stretching.

Up to 30 percent of your propulsive power comes from the energy stored when you land on each stride – you convert the energy coming in on landing, store it in your muscles and tendons instead of wasting the energy. Keep your muscles strong and elastic with weight training and stretching respectively.

Muscles are 10 percent shorter than normal when you wake up; 10 percent longer than average for the day after warming up. So...do your stretches with warm muscles, and stretch gently. Muscles work better when they are long, exerting the same force with less effort: flexibility will improve your running.

Doing one stretch for each muscle group is sufficient; do each stretch 2 to 3 times and hold each stretch for 15 to 30 seconds.

Stretching reflex. Near the junction of tendon to muscle lie muscle spindles and Golgi tendon organs (proprioceptors) which initiate the tendon-muscle reflex to prevent muscles from lengthening too far. When muscle tension is too high, the muscle is not allowed beyond a certain length. Hold a steady stretch for 20 seconds, and this deep myotatic reflex eases...your muscle is allowed to go one or two percent longer...so hold a stretch, then seek a little extra pain free elongation after 20-30 seconds.

Calf Muscles: stand 3 to 4 feet from a wall or sturdy support.

Put your outstretched hands on the wall, shoulder width apart. Keep the knees straight and the heels flat on the ground. Lean in toward the wall slowly, keeping the body and knees straight: Stop when you think the calf muscles are at their limit...when they and the Achilles tendons feel stretched. This stretches the gastrocnemious, the large muscle close to your skin.

Next, to emphasize the soleus muscle which lies under the gastroc, stand as above but 2 to 3 feet away. Bend the knees until you feel the stretch and again, keep your heels on the ground.

Or, do this pictured version.

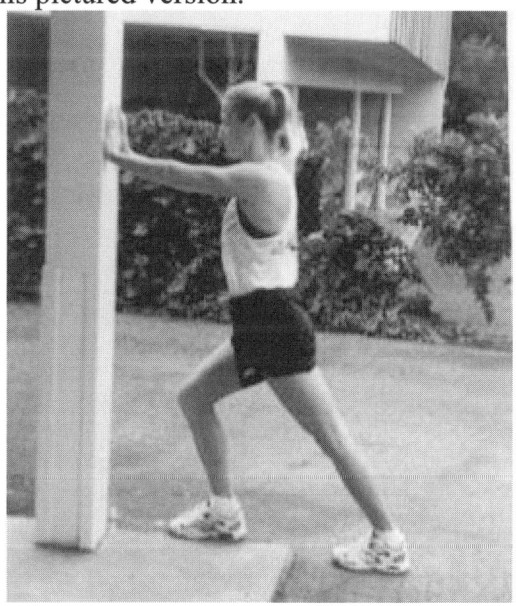

Quadriceps: the front of the thigh. Stand upright, hold one foot
and pull it toward your bottom. Keep the knee pointed down. Or to make sure the Iliacus and psoas muscles get stretched, place one leg well behind you on a support. Move forward as if into a lunge while staying tall and feel the stretch at the front of your hips.

Hamstrings: back of the thigh. Sit on a soft surface, keep the
knees straight and bend forward at the waist. Move your head down toward the knees or beyond. Or...stand on one leg and place the other foot on a support at knee height or a bit higher. Role around the hip joint to give slight tension to the hamstring.

Hip extensor muscles (buttock or gluteal muscles): Lie on
your back on a comfortable surface. Grasp one leg at the shin; pull
the knee up toward your chest.

I-T band (or Ileotibial Band): As above, but then bring
the left knee across the chest toward your right armpit; then re-
stretch it toward the right side of your pelvis. Do the other leg too.

Trunk: Stand with your feet apart; keep your hips facing the
front. Bend over to one side as far as possible...hold, and do the
other side. Next, from the standing position, rotate the top of the
trunk to look behind. Keep the hips facing forward...hold; swing
slowly around to the front...and to the other side.

   For the lower back, butt muscles and hamstrings: Feet
together or apart, knees bent or straight...bend over and ease your
hands toward your feet. Just hang loose; let the tension go but
don't force it. Or do it sitting on the floor.

Calf, gluts and hamstrings are partial to the walk your
fingers to your feet pictured on page 43. Start in the standing
position with your feet facing forward, but about 30 inches apart.
Hang your arms down and relax your back. Bend your knees as
you place your hands on the floor in front of you...well in front of
you. Straighten your legs; locked knees are not essential. Your butt
should be well into the air. Now, walk your hands back toward
your toes. Hold, relax per usual, and then get a little closer to your
toes as you improve flexibility. Walk back on your fingers if you
need too. You have just done yoga's downward-facing dog.

   If you do it in a yoga class, you'll be on hands and knees and
then raise your butt into the air while straightening your knees and
keeping your heels on the ground.

   Downward dog beats the shoulder press according to an article
in August 2,004s Fitness Magazine. It's a great way to stretch and
exercise the shoulders, while also stretching your calves and
hamstrings.

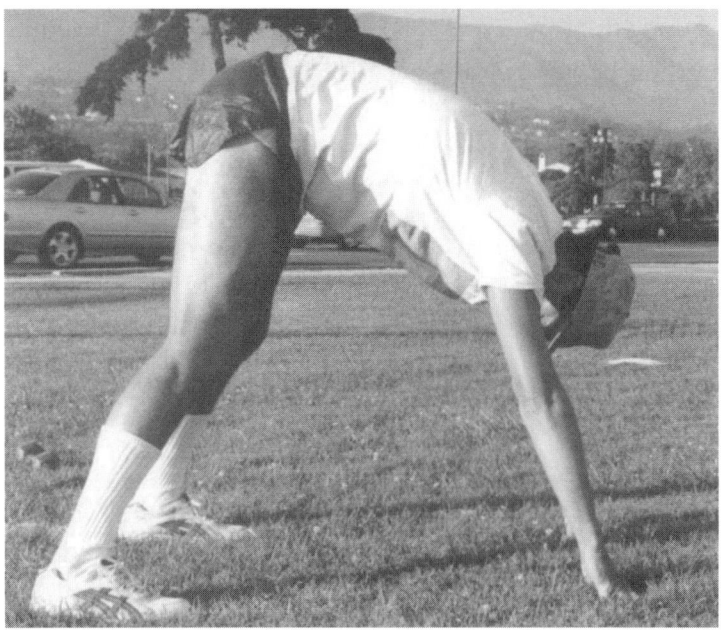

Shoulders are too far from the knees to qualify as downward dog, but he is getting a nice stretch for the calves and hammies. Based on the tree growing out of his rear he is consuming enough fiber.

Yoga offers many other stretching and muscle strengthening options. Take a few beginner yoga classes, but don't stretch too far or you'll get injured. Do some of the static balance drills at home using a yoga tape or DVD.

Example: The tree. Stand tall with arms at your side and weight evenly balanced on your feet. Slowly lift one foot along your inner leg toward your thigh. Raise your arms to the side for balance as your weight bearing leg makes constant adjustments to keep you standing. If your balance is up to it, place your hands together at your chest. Hold for 20-30 seconds and breathe slowly, and then do it with the other leg. Later, raise your arms above your head to expand the lungs.

Stay in balance with a stretching routine and you'll be less injury prone. Sadly, stretching is the third leading cause of running injuries. Stretch with warm muscles and stretch gently. Stretching just after a shower is better than immediately after a tough run. Think relaxation and visualize pleasant surroundings such as a beach, lake or the mountains as you ease through your stretches.

You can try progressive relaxation in addition to stretching. Lie down. Gently tense your hand muscles and maintain tension for 5 to 7 seconds then relax; then tense your arm muscles and move through the entire body a muscle group at a time to finish with your feet. If you have oodles of time, do your dominant side followed by your less active or less coordinated side.

Never stretch in an elevator. I've seen time saver hints to stretch in these fine machines, yet pressure changes are sudden as you stop and start from floor to floor, which stimulates a strained muscle.

amtamassage.org will help you find a massage therapist if you knead more help in relaxing your muscles.

Back to the running.

Subsequent runs should follow every other day until you can run easily, the distance which you used to walk in 40 minutes. Use several routes to avoid boredom. When you feel ready to increase your run, add a loop to your present course...or use an out and back system. Run for half of your intended running time away from the start point, and aim to run back in the same time.

Increase the time of your run by a few minutes at a time, as shown in Chapter One, but get used to your new level before moving on. When you can manage thirty minutes at a time, consider training on consecutive days...once and then twice a week. Your target is to run five times a week, but for different periods. Shorter runs will be rest days between the longish runs.

As you get fitter, you'll notice things in your area such as hidden paths and plants. Be kind to strolling pedestrians; you'll soon be moving three times faster than them. No weaving in and out. Use quiet streets because busy streets upset your rhythm. Make eye contact with pedestrians and motorists to help you decide which way they are going.

In due course, your training should look something like this.
Saturday – 30 minutes paths and grass
Sun – 20 mins road
Mon – 30 mins road & park
Tue – rest
Wed – 30 mins road
Th – 20 mins grass
Fri – rest

To repeat a theme, the actual days that you run is a personal choice based on convenience and logic. Fridays or Sundays huge religious days for you? They are probably not the best days for exercise.

For variety, run in areas with different terrain. Use several road and path circuits and find some grass. Grass should be short so that you can see the holes. Golf course fairways near sunrise or dusk are good. Holes 10 to 18 are usually empty for the first hour of daylight. Holes one to nine are often empty in the last hour before sunset. In summer, these are also the best times of day to run!

Use the edge of a park if it's over half a mile around the outside. Larger parks and woods are better for steady runs as you'll have fewer laps to run. Run on wide dirt trails to avoid holes.

Run on flat surfaces. Avoid sloped beaches, banked indoor tracks, or cambered roads, which make your feet roll too much. Avoid concrete because it's six times harder than asphalt, and avoid the jarring from going up and down sidewalks. The soft sand at the top of a beach can be perfect for strength training. Your heels will drop down on every stride giving your calves and Achilles a good stretch; you'll also have to push off harder with those calf muscles. Landing softly will let your skeleton strengthen at its own pace.

Run at appropriate pace and you'll find that regular exercise is more relaxing than a laxative...or was it sedative.

<u>Slightly Overweight?</u> Get used to people looking at you in admiration as you take your overweight or out of shape body through gentle walking or running at a heartrate of 120 to 150 beats per minute. Feel admired, not embarrassed by people looking at you. You are "doing it" to paraphrase one sports company, they are not exercising.

You can still hide in aqua-aerobics classes if you wish, or go to grassy areas, high school tracks after the team has practiced and fitness clubs mid-morning or early afternoon to enjoy anonymity while exercising because few people are there to watch. Any person who shouts an insult to you is actually insulting himself!

Switch to shorts when you feel ready. Overcome your perceived obstacles or excuses to get fit for life and give yourself a sporting chance of seeing your grand-children grow up.

Chapter Four

On ANIMALS, WEATHER, CLOTHS & HEARTRATEs

Coping with dogs.

Although running on grass and paths is better for your legs, it tends to bring you into frequent contact with man's best friend. When running on roads and sidewalks, you seldom come across dogs without their pets. Alas, when dogs enter a park, woods, or a recreation ground, they usually let their pets off the leash, to sit down for a rest, or amble around...perhaps throwing sticks or balls to assist the dog in its exercise session.

Part of this session may involve chasing you. Sometimes it seems as if each dog you meet would like to take a bite out of your lean, muscular legs. Most dogs will either ignore you or look up from their ball chasing activities to wish you an enjoyable run. A few, however, will take chase, or run at full speed to meet a runner.

The dog is having fun, then some stranger comes charging toward her. It's not surprising if some dogs dislike this intrusion.

To decrease the dogs' fear of attack, give her a wide birth when possible. Veer away from her at 45 to 60 degrees.

Slowing down will reassure her also. If she still shows interest in you...stop. Say something reassuring to her. Talk as if to a friend, at a neutral volume. Don't smile...showing your teeth signals aggression to many animals. And don't look her directly in the eyes because that is a form of challenging her.

You can also pick up a small rock or stick or just pretend to do so. Throw the stick away from both of you to see what happens; or pretend to throw something at her: if all else fails, actually throw something at her.

Only shout at her if she's about to attack you. Provided she is wagging her tail, and perhaps looking playful, you should be safe. If the hairs on the back of its neck are standing up, and talking has not calmed her down, withdrawing is required. Move away while facing the dog: don't give her a clear shot at your rear.

Most runners believe in friendship. In this situation, a runner can simply get down on one knee and call the dog to them. This thwarts any cunning the dog might have used. Many dogs come quietly up to the kneeling runner. The dog no longer feels threatened, so she doesn't feel the need to threaten you. Some dogs will scamper back to their pets. A few will still give the impression that they want to fight. One or two are very difficult to gauge.

Here are a couple of incidents which show how his advice works. I did a run in a different part of town. "Neighborhood Watch," read the sign...should be safe from burglary here I thought. Well, every house seemed to posses barking dogs. Some were behind fences, a couple chained at the front, and finally of course...loose dogs: Three of them.

I was unsure about the six month pup; it was barring its teeth a little too much. However, the other two, though barking, seemed friendly enough. When I got down and called them to me, one just ran back to the house. A second came up to be stroked, and then joined his companion. The pup slinked round at an angle, about 60 degrees from my front.

I faced him again, slapped my thigh, and held out my hand (palm downwards) for him to smell. I talked soothingly to him. "Come here, you seething mass of over-aggressive, retarded piece of protoplasm." Not being a linguist...he complied. It took several minutes for me to calm this skittish pup enough to be able to stand up and back away. I probably should have used this next approach.

Later in the run, I came to the back of a property from which three inviting trails led off. Frost would have been proud of me because I ran up the most inviting of those trails. After a few hundred yards, I saw two dogs coming at a modest tempo toward me. Their intent was clear. My reaction was swift. Outrunning never being an option with dogs, I turned and walked back from whence I came. Perhaps because I was moving away from "their" property, they slowed somewhat. When the lead dog was 45 feet away, I used my firmest no-nonsense shout, "Stay." It had the desired effect. After I'd walked another 30 yards, I resumed running.

I've since found the one syllable approach to be the best. "No," works quite well.

You'll often find the dog's pet reading while the dog chases you. Their most likely comment is, "she won't bite."

Request its owner to restrain it. Some dogs will chase runners all the time. If talking to its pet fails, consider the next step. Find out the owner's name and then walk away from the area. Generally, you should walk away while facing the animal. Having walked out of chasing range, resume your run.

The dog clearly has a right to exercise, but by Law it must be kept under control. If you have a problem with one or more dogs in an area, a word with the Police Dept or animal control may help. They, or you, can get a restraining order requiring the dog to be kept under control. If a dog bites you, report this to animal control. Although a dog usually gets more than one bite before its life is in danger, the first report ought to remind the owner of his duty to keep it under control.

Shouting at the dog is of use in an actual attack, as is the aptly named Halt spray, which has saved many lives. Mace and pepper sprays are also effective. Inexpensive, they are easily attached to shorts or carried in the hand. Halt is a key part of running gear.

As you add a couple of minutes to the length of some runs each week, your training will move toward this.

Saturday – 40 minutes paths and grass
Sun – 30 mins road
Mon – 30 mins road & park
Tue – rest
Wed – 40 mins trails and road
Th – 30 mins grass
Fri – rest

Now that you're close to the three hour per week threshold, let's consider other things. Many people think running is a cheap sport: Then they find out how expensive shoes, weather suits and sundry equipment cost. However, it needn't cost the earth. All you need is a little protection from the ground (shoes) and the elements (clothing).

Footwear, AKA Running Shoes

For the first few weeks, one pair of running shoes should meet all of your needs. However, they require several qualities. In addition to being comfortable, they need enough cushioning to protect you from the shock of landing on a hard surface thousands of times on each run. To help traction on wet grass and paths they will need a sole with waffles, ripples and or studs.

Running shoes absorb much of the shock from landing on the ground. You can reduce your shoes workload by running on grass and dirt whenever possible and by taking short strides and landing with a slightly flexed knee.

Let them dry naturally or with an assist from a fan, but not close to a heat source, and not in harsh sunlight. Dirty shoes are fine; scrap the worst of the mud off but don't ruin them by putting them in the washer let alone the drier. Shoes lose resiliency when wet, which is fine if you're running on sand flats covered by 3 inches of water. However, if you're cruising packed trails, try to avoid *running* through the river crossings until the last mile. Don't use running shoes for court games.

Stability shoes are for the majority of runners who have normal feet.

Motion control shoes are quite rigid to reduce the joint movements within the foot. Motion control shoes keep your foot stable and especially support the medial or inner side of your fragile limb. This type of shoe is vital for flat footed (who often overpronate) and heavy runners.

The cushioned shoe belongs to high arched people. Runners with high arches don't usually pronate very much. There feet don't absorb much of the ground shock either. Motion control and stability shoes do contain plenty of cushioning. However, the cushioned shoe encourages your feet to pronate a more reasonable amount, which will improve your running gait and efficiency.

Have a podiatrist, coach or an experienced runner watch your running form, or get yourself video taped. Experts in running shoe stores can be your best specialists. Show them your first pair of running shoes and test run a few new pairs while they watch.

Like the podiatrist, you can check your old shoes to see your running type:

Shoe wear on the outer heel, the ball of the foot and the front of the sole is a normal wear pattern which is characteristic of normal feet and economical running.

If you overpronate, the shoe wear will be more to the inside edge of each shoe, and the inside edge may be compressed too.

The underpronator usually has a wear pattern to the outer part of the shoe from heel to forefoot.

You can do an additional test at home. Walk a few steps with bare feet and then place them about 3 inches apart. The normal feet possessed by about 50 percent of people will be directly below the knees. The big toes will point forward. You are a neutral runner, and your feet should roll nicely or pronate about the right amount. You probably will not need an anti-pronation or anti-supination shoe, but you still have three choices based on measuring the length of your feet when sitting and standing.

* No change? Your feet are rigid and you'll probably get a good ride from cushioned shoes.
* Foot length increase by 3 millimeters or less when you stand up, makes you a normal, normal. (Normal pronation and normal flexibility.) Seems weird, but your shoe type is a stability shoe.
* Highly flexible feet increase in length by more than 3 millimeters and while stability shoes work for many, a motion-control shoe is appreciated by others.

About one quarter of peoples' feet splay outward when standing (called duck feet by some). Arches usually collapse during impact shock, which can wreak havoc on your Achilles, shins, knees and hips. Your shoe type is clearly a stability or motion control for overpronators, and most of your mileage should probably be on board lasted or combination lasted shoes. There are racing shoes and performance trainers for overpronators. Orthotics allow many runners to use cushioned or regular running shoes.

Wear anti-pronation shoes if appropriate. Different pronators need different amounts of resistance on the inside to stop their feet from rolling over. Just because your pronating friend swears by his 'Ni-bok' 220s, doesn't mean they'll suit you. Based on advertisements you would think that 90 percent of runners overpronate, but you're only about 25 percent of the running population. If your shoes are bashed in on the inside after a couple of hundred miles, you need a meatier anti-pronation device and possibly orthotics, but you can also work on running form.

Roughly another one quarter of peoples' <u>feet splay inward</u> in the standing test, which is pigeon toed. You have a tendency toward high arches and rigid feet which <u>underpronate</u> on each stride, decreasing your ability to absorb shock. You'll need extra cushioning and perhaps a single-density midsole. A curved last or a slip lasted base will assist your cushioning, making them soft and flexible which encourages you to pronate a bit. You may also be called <u>supinators</u> because you land on the inner part of the foot and then roll outwards, though many of you are partial to landing on the outer part of the foot (anywhere from heel to little toe) but not pronating or rolling over enough.

The <u>wet foot test</u> is another predictor of your arches' habits. With wet feet, stand on a few sheets of newspaper, and then check your foot's shape.
* If you see your entire arch in your foot-print, you have a low flexible arch or flat foot, and you'll probably overpronate.
* If you see almost nothing of the arch in your foot-print, you're high arched and likely to underpronate.
* Have a foot-print which is not as wide in the middle of the foot than at the heel? You're lucky and some would say you're normal! You should have a neutral foot plant in running because you have medium arches.

All runners should <u>buy their shoes late in the day</u>, when feet have expanded to their largest point. Wear your normal running socks and your orthotics to test them. Get your feet measured. Your shoes will need to be about half an inch beyond your big toe…when you're standing. The forefoot needs space for its movement too. Buy for the largest foot. If you need to, add padding or an extra sock to your small foot. Wear a size 9 running shoe? Some manufacturers may be a half size or more either way. Test them. You'll need a snug fit at the heel to prevent slipping on every stride, but the ball of your foot needs comfort too. After checking comfort with walking, take a few hundred yards of running to give the final test. Therefore, don't go shopping a few hours after your longest run of the week. Just like mobile homes, running shoes come double and triple wide; their widths vary considerably.

Overpronator or not,

your feet may roll at different rates, so the wonkiest foot needs correcting. Stop that one from wobbling on each stride, and the better foot's workload is also lessened. Heed the store-person's advice but give a nod to how each shoe feels to you. Arch supports or orthotics inside the shoe may also be needed.

If only your right foot overpronates, running with the traffic will allow the camber to correct your body's fault. However, long term, it is better to get your footwear corrected by using orthotics so that you can run on a variety of flat surfaces, plus you won't have to trust drivers to avoid you.

Orthotics or a simple heel lift one side can also adjust your leg length differences, which reduces the strain on your longest leg. Note: it is usually your longest leg which gets injured.

Avoid the expensive shoes with special devices. A mid priced, but robust shoe from one of the major shoe makers such as Asics, Nike or New Balance will do for starters. If it becomes apparent from the way your shoes wear down that you have a problem, you can consider other options.

Your shoes may last 500 miles if you're lucky. When they are half-way to wearing out, consider specializing. A second pair for runs on asphalt is useful. Then alternate the shoes as you alternate the terrain you run on. As the months role by you can relegate old running shoes for your cycling and weight training sessions, while rotating two or three pairs of fresh shoes for your running.

The three or four day break between runs allow the materials in the shoe to get back to normal after being compressed during your run, and to dry out. Using different shoes also reduces repetitive stress syndrome, which can hurt your muscles and joints.

www.runnersworld.com has an up to date shoe guide. Runner's World magazine's April and October issue has its routine reviews. Big 5 and other chain stores generally have several pairs at half-price, and will sell most of last years shoe designs at a discount.

This author sees no point in using special running socks because their seams are no better than a decent sport sock from a department store. A six pack of department store white socks with cushioning cost about the same as one pair of "running socks." When you've broken in your shoes properly and provided you don't suddenly run 5 miles more than usual, you should only get blisters if you leave a ridge of sock in your shoe. While you can get synthetic running socks which wick moisture away from your skin, they are just as likely to ridge and blister you.

Clean the blisters you do get with soap and water before applying antibiotic lotion and covering with a non stick dressing. You may still need to soak the dressing off 24 hours later to avoid taking off the healing tissue with it. Keep using the antibiotic until you're healed and put a thin layer between the blister site and your sock in future runs if you're prone to blisters. Vaseline, bodyglide or antiperspirants also decreases blister risk over trouble spots.

If you tend to blister or chaff at the armpits, groin or nipples, use gels and lotions for comfort and prevention. Vaseline, topped by a bandaid will protect the nipples. Females can top that with a comfortable sports bra to control most of the bounce. With the improvement in support offered by bra tops, many A and B sized people get sufficient stability without a sports bra.

Shorts and stuff.

Hot days and cold days should rarely prevent you from running. What clothing you wear when running will depend on the time of year, the training effort you intend to put in, and your personal feelings. Runners who want to look good, will need a couple of multicolored track suits or sweats, and a Gore-Tex, breathable waterproof to put in their closet. They won't actually run in the rain because it would mess their attire and ruin the coffee house look.

The main thing is to stay warm. Shorts, lightweight and normal thickness track bottoms all have their uses depending on the conditions. With the advent of the built-in supportive liner to running shorts, the jock strap should have faded from manufacturing 25 years ago. A good supply of T-shirts and sweatshirts of various thicknesses will take care of the trunk. For wet days, you will need a lightweight, shower-proof jacket and possibly trousers. Take great care when wearing these, because you can easily overheat.

When the temperature is low, do wrap up well. Gloves and hat are usually required at some stage of the winter. You can use mittens and inner linings on really cold days, or add hand warmer gels which act like a warm compress when you've pre-heated them or mixed the chemicals in the bag. Check outdoor and mountain retailers. The outer garment should be wind and water resistant. When you're increasing the length of your run, use circuits close to a warm base. On windy days, a forest will give you shelter, but it will also stay frosty for longer than areas where the sun has had a chance to work. Houses can give you good shelter too if you choose a street which is at right angles to the wind's direction.

When running an out and back route, usually start into the wind; you'll then be pushed back to your start point in the second half of the run, decreasing the possibility of getting chilled. Running back into the wind with tired legs makes the session feel harder. When you are well experienced, you can run a long warm-up with the wind, followed by a harder effort into the wind on the way back.

Any day that you overheat, take the top sweatshirt off and tie it around your waist. If you feel warm early in the run, stop to adjust what you're wearing. You can stash the extra gear to pick up on the way back. Your hat is the easiest temperature regulator, so take it off as required.

At the start of a run you should feel cool but not cold. If your indoor warmup exercises make you feel toasty when you step out of the door, you're probably wearing too much.

Clothing should wick the perspiration away from the skin, to the outer layer, so that it can evaporate. You perspire to lose heat. Excessive sweating during a winter run would suggest you're wearing too much. If all this sweat is allowed to stay trapped on the skin, the exerciser could get too cold, especially if he stops exercising or decreases the rate at which he exercises.

It's difficult to figure out how many layers to wear for certain conditions. A small, waterproof fanny pack, with a long sleeve T-shirt, is useful. If conditions worsen, you can use it as an extra layer. If you start too fast, or if you've slowed down and begin to feel cold, you can exchange the dry one for the inner, wet shirt you had on for the first part of the run. Then head back to your base at a pace that won't make you sweat up too much. The inner layer should be like a diaper lining, able to make you feel dry for hours.

The outer, waterproof layer should be breathable to allow moisture to escape. Don't put too much heavy stuff underneath because you shouldn't be sweating like you would in summer.

There is no product which allows that amount of moisture out. Dress to lightly perspire, not to sweat.

Running at low temperatures or in wet weather doesn't give you pneumonia, flu or colds: people do. Rain and snow harbor no virus or bacteria. The hand you shake after a good run probably does have nastiness on it, especially if it's owner cleared his nose in the standard way. That said, do get some dry clothes on once you've finished the run so that you stay warm. Then, if you've been running with company or met someone on your route, go and wash your hands to get rid of his or her germs!

For wet spells, you'll need at least two pairs of shoes to avoid starting runs with yesterday's wet shoes. After wet runs, take the inserts and orthotics out. Squeeze out excessive moisture then pack the shoe with scrunched up newspaper and change it three of four times at 60 minute intervals. Place the shoes in a warm spot but away from heaters and direct sunlight. A fan will speed the drying if you STILL only have one pair.

On hot days, you'll take almost the opposite clothing approach. Your muscles produce huge amounts of heat as a byproduct of repeated contractions and you must learn to dissipate the heat with minimal sweating: don't overdress.

Loose fitting, lightweight and light colored materials will reflect the sun instead of absorbing more heat and allow maximum heat loss. Expose goodly amounts of sun-blocked skin for maximum heat loss. Run with the wind in the first half of the run and enjoy the cooling breeze running into the wind on your return.

To complete your getup, you should buy a runner or cyclist bib to help motorists see you. This needs a bright eye-catching *fluorescent* part for daylight recognition, and a *reflective* part for nighttime. It's up to you to make yourself visible and therefore safer on the roads. As a runner, you are probably more alert than the 85,000 pedestrians per year injured in traffic related incidents in the United States. Rely on all of your senses though and leave the musical device at home. Use roads mainly as a way of getting to paths, tracks and grass where most of your running can take place.

Some people think that roads belong to engined vehicles. Having dressed to be seen, remember to keep your eyes and ears open for them. Keep to the sidewalk if there are only a few cross streets; face oncoming traffic if there's no sidewalk. On rural roads, it may be safer to switch sides when traffic is only coming from one direction. When the curves are as tight as a lingerie models, drivers won't see even a brightly clad runner until nearly upon you. If you hear it in time, pop across the road; he will see you earlier, and he won't have to move out to avoid you.

At night, if you close one eye when a car approaches you'll retain some of your night vision.

A flashing red light on a belt, or shoes that flash are useful aids to being seen. A small flashlight with a strong beam also helps you to be seen, and helps you to see hazards ahead.

When running at night, keep to known routes and you'll have a better idea of the hazards. Be even more careful with curbs and cross-streets. Late night and early morning running means the metal manhole covers are more likely to be wet. Take a shorter stride before touching down on these slippery surfaces and don't try to push off hard or accelerate across them. Don't strain your hamstrings by jumping over them either.

Run with a higher knee lift at night, which will raise your feet above many objects and surface imperfections. Land soft...ready to allow your leg to fold partially if the surface surprises you...prepare to fall and roll.

Street lights can help, but they're likely to lead you through heavily vehicled and therefore polluted areas. Running indoors is an option for many, though once or twice a week is most people's limit. The speed sessions in Chapter Seven work well on a treadmill.

Don't wear a musical device. While reasonably safe to use at a populated track (at least ten people actively exercising...giving all present some degree of safety) or on an indoor exercise machine, music listeners still need to stay out of the inner lanes, avoid changing lanes suddenly, and look before changing lanes to remain safe. Warning: Tracks can empty quite rapidly; you have to set your own safety limit.

The second reason to avoid musical devices is that there are too many noisy intrusions on your auditory system as it is. Give your mind a break and take in the silence. Listen to the background churning of your brain and think your own random thoughts for thirty to forty minutes.

Exercise Intensity & Heartrate Goals.

Most of you athletes (yes that's you, an athlete) should avoid running hills for the first few weeks, but you can then introduce them into some of your runs to get used to the slightly different running action they require. Don't go for anything too demanding, but include a few hills in new routes you plan. Get used to running them economically. Shorten your stride length a bit; if necessary, reduce the leg speed also. Shuffle up with a low knee lift and a relaxed lower arm action. If you get very short of breath, stop and resume at a slower pace.

Hills will slow down your running pace. As with running itself, you may take several attempts to find the right speed for each gradient and length of hill. The aim should be to run well within yourself and accelerate to your normal pace over the top. In the fullness of time you will get your leg speed back when moving up-hill and develop more legspeed when running downhills. At this early stage, stay at the same heartrate on your hilly sections.

Coaches generally accept the talk test as the simplest indication of the speed to run at, in order to gain significant training benefit. There are many other ways to assess ideal running pace, with your "training effort" confirmed by simple formulae. The starting point for this one is your heartrate at rest (an indicator or current fitness).

(200 - pulse at rest) x 60 % + pulse at rest

Examples

Heartrate at rest 80:

200 - 80 = 120

120 x 60 % = 72

72 + 80 gives a heartrate of 152 to be maintained throughout the run.

Pulse at rest	target in run
70	148
60	144
50	140
40	136

Other formulae take account of age. Most reduce by one, the target pulse for each year above a certain age: Thirty is the usual starting age. A fifty-year-old with a pulse at rest of 70 would have his target pulse reduced to 128. As you become fitter, this age allowance is reduced until you enjoy the same target as a thirty-year-old. Use the target only as a guide because the talk test is the most important at this stage.

For the time being, check your pulse five minutes before the end of a run. Do this is on a flat section, and don't increase your speed before the heartrate check or it will give you a false reading. Just stop running...count your pulse for ten seconds while walking, then resume running at a slower pace to finish the run. This gives you a nice warmdown.

The number of beats in ten seconds, times six, will give a fairly accurate figure. Try to be within 12 beats either way of your target. More than 12 beats per minute above target, and you're really doing a Chapter 7 or 8 type run. More than 12 below may not be giving you sufficient stimulation for your endurance to improve.

Once every few weeks, carry out the pulse or heartrate test at the ten and twenty minute stage of a few runs. You may be starting out too fast and slowing down after 20 minutes!

Another way to recognize you started out too fast is if YOU hear your feet hitting the pavement. It can indicate that your form has broken down. Walk for a minute, and then get your running form back at a slower pace. If you're able to talk in 8 to 10 word sentences without huffing and puffing...you're at the right pace.

Heartrate monitors make checking HR easier of course, and there are reliable models for around $60. Expensive ones require you to be a Ph.D. candidate to use all of their functions; though computer downloading of minute by minute heartrates does make some runners happy, maximum heartrate on a particular run and the average heartrate for your run is all that you really need.

Unless you're doing speed training, the max on a particular run should only be 75 percent of your actual maximum heartrate. Glance at your monitor at the end of a few reps during speed training to check your intensity. As you'll see in Chapters 7 and 8, 85 to 90 percent of max heartrate is the goal during tempo running. During Chapters 10 and 11, 95 to 98 percent of max heartrate is your goal. Use a monitor for half of your runs and rely upon yourself and your breathing on the other runs. Heartrate Monitor sources include:

1. Chain sports stores such as Big 5.
2. www.cardiosport.com

3.   www.timex.com
4.   www.polarusa.com

Believe in yourself and you can achieve great things, including fitness. Believe you can run for 40 minutes, and provided you add only a couple of minutes to your runs every week or two, you will soon reach your goal of 40 minute runs.

Keep a training diary to see how your fitness progresses. A grade school composition notebook works well. One page per week gives you two and a half years of exercise memories.

When you've achieved the 40 minute goal, increase your pace to run at 65, then 70 and 75 percent of max heartrate with one run each week at each intensity level.

Many weeks of 40 minute runs give you endurance for life and the strength to move onto the quality running of the next few chapters. Progress may have seemed slow at first, yet you're:

o   Off of the sofa 5 days a week;
o   You've already decreased your risk from over a dozen diseases, and;
o   You're about to start more entertaining types of running.

Running Safety

Run with someone if you're in unfamiliar surroundings, or when running in the dark. While daylight running is safer (including a lower potential for tripping up), night running is generally safe if:

*   You stay away from undesirable areas such as where the homeless gather or run-down places.
*   Monitor alleys and corners.
*   Don't run to exhaustion. Muggers can spot a tired runner just as easily as a lion spots the weak antelope! Look pooped or demoralized and you're an instant target.
*   Run tall and look confident.
*   Do your stretches and clothing changes in safe places.
*   Use the track safety rule. More than 10 people present and moving with a definite purpose and you're probably safe.
*   Nearly empty running tracks or streets are an attackers dream.
*   Beware of your quiet neighborhood. Vary your routes to be unpredictable.
*   Don't wear flashy cloths or reveal expensive gadgets.

* Never run with a musical device. You need all of your senses.
* In addition, carry pepper spray or Halt in an easily accessible position.
* An opportunistic drive-by attack upon your body or your equipment is just that...opportunistic.

Lyme Disease

This annoying "non plague" is not a serious danger to runners, but it's useful to know a bit about what the bacterium does and how it is transferred. Lyme does not kill...but if untreated, it's unhealthy for you. The disease has been in the U.S. for at least a century.

Deer do not give people Lyme, but the deer tick is the carrier of the bacteria for Lyme. A Deer tick feeds only once a year and is unlikely to give Lyme to you.

The tick takes about 24 hours to cement itself to you...then it will take a blood meal. If you live or run in Lyme country, check your body twice a day for ticks, stay on trails, wear white to easily spot the ticks, and enjoy your running. Don't roll around in the grass in Lyme country. Wear tights or sweats over your legs while walking or running grassy trails.

Few states have more than a hundred cases of Lyme Disease each year. What if you're one of those who get it?

A bull's-eye shaped rash (*erythema migrans*), of several inches diameter and flu symptoms are typical signs.

Confirmation is by a simple blood test. Treatment is easy and successful provided you take your antibiotics correctly.

Attorney Avoidance.

Snakes are not dangerous, unless you're allergic to their poison or you habitually play with them. Most people bitten by snakes don't even receive venom or venin; most who receive it can get to an antivenin source before it causes damage.

If you're allergic to the venom however, you could go into anaphylactic shock; unless you have expert assistance, you'll be one of the 20 or so in the U.S. who die from snake-bites...out of 45,000 bitten.

Bees aren't dangerous either, though they may be high in your psyche if you just found out that they kill three to five times more people than snakes in the United States...and you're being chased by a swarm because they liked your sweet running aroma.

Give beehives a wide birth. If you're the one in two hundred who is allergic to stings, always carry your epinephrine.

As your running speed increases by a few seconds per mile, it becomes even more important to cooldown or warmdown at the end of your sessions. Though no studies have proven a lower injury risk without cooling down, a cooldown of 5 minutes at slower pace does make you feel as if the main part of the run was easier.

You'll also decrease stiffness, end with a pleasant feeling, and you're more likely to run again the next day.

The next few chapters show many types of speed running. Avoid speedy running at the end of sessions. Always finish with 5 to 10 minutes at steady pace.

Get your sleep.

As you'll see in Appendix I, regular exercise increases your chances of getting quality sleep, though it will not do so unless you give it the opportunity.

Your muscles need physical rest to get stronger. Exercise will wear you out if your muscle fibers are left fatigued for weeks at a time. Get 7 to 9 hours sleep per night, especially mid-week nights because research shows that you will not catch up at the weekend. Get decent amounts of sleep during your vacations too so that you come back rested.

Exercise while on vacation: Don't do the same old exercise when on vacation, but do some exercise. See the area you're purported to be visiting by running the parks or trails. Check a map and carry safety gear such as water and a windproof jacket. Long run each week 10 miles at 9-minute miles? Aim for 8 miles at 9.30 pace to save your legs for the museums.

To avoid having to take off the weight on your return, moderate your consumption of calorie containing liquids. Eat mostly healthful foods in modest quantities too, while sampling the local delights.

Chapter Five

STYLE AND SPEED
with
ONE HUNDREDS & FARTLEK

Periodization of training is a cutesy phrase which coaches use to say that you'll spend a period of time specializing in new types of training in several phases to get stronger, faster and fitter. The training phases build upon each other to give you a well rounded fitness. The next two chapters bring in faster running and strength running. You'll develop speed gently to avoid strains: your running style or running form will change slightly as you become more efficient. Three different sessions will be brought into your schedule.

The more time you spend running, the more important good running form is for reducing your injury potential. Good form also improves your use of the limited oxygen supply. The best mechanical efficiency for you, which generally means *smooth* running, means more enjoyable running and faster races.

These are not sprinting sessions and don't think of them as speedwork. Anything with work in its structure creates negative feelings. Fast running is play at its best. Watch a few puppies chase each other, they'll stop, check out a few smells while recovering, and then chase again. You'll be doing the same as a puppy or child, one of which you were several to many years ago.

Physical stress reduces mental stress...provided the physical stress is mild enough. Actually, physical stress or exercise only helps you to cope with mental stress. The act of finding the time to exercise, plus the exercise itself, takes you out of the stress cycle. Your anxiety level will stay down longer after exercise if you do some of it at moderate intensity with striders or 3 to 15 minutes at over 80 percent of your maximum heartrate as in Chapters 7 & 8. Don't allow this quicker exercise to add stress to your life.

So, make no sudden changes in training. Keep your speed sessions fun; they should not be intense. When possible, do them in natural surroundings.

As your heart, lungs and leg muscles now have a solid foundation of steady running, you can move onto faster running. Provided you can manage several thirty minute runs a week, you can introduce one session of this fast running per week. On reaching the magic forty minute run without aches and pains, you can increase to two speed sessions per week.

Although an untrained person can sprint for a bus, it's unwise to run fast until you have first trained slowly. Endurance must come first. You can then use this phase or period of running to build more endurance while also playing at speed.

Fast running adds to your strength and endurance. Running moderately fast in short sections is good stimulation and will not over stress the body: it allows your body to work harder. You gain very quick results from running short distances many times within a session. You will still do a steady run on alternate training days.

The heart, being a muscle, also improves. The muscle itself becomes larger and stronger. Each heartbeat pumps out more blood. We call this the stroke volume. Stroke volume multiplied by your heartrate is your cardiac output. All very nice of course, so here's the nitty gritty: Steady training and striders will increase your stroke volume and therefore your cardiac output by 25 percent, sending greater amounts of oxygen enriched blood to your running muscles.

Choose a quiet area for your first speed session. Use about 100 meters of reasonably flat and even grass. After warming up with ten minutes of easy running, do your stretches and then discard the outer layer of gear or clothing. Stride out a little faster than normal...progressively build your speed. Do not sprint. Maintain fairly good speed for about 50 meters then ease off or decelerate. Walk a few meters until your breathing is easy, and then repeat the stride back to your gear.

You should aim for about ten minutes of these strides and work up to the full 100 meters at speed. As the weeks progress, experiment with your running style. See what happens when you work your arms harder, or pick your knees up a little higher, or take short, quite rapid strides.

Don't get too much out of breath at first. Enjoy the session, and use it as an appetizer for the next one.

You're looking for smoothness in your running: avoid jerky movements. The smooth, economic runner will use less oxygen at a given speed, and will be able to run faster for every liter of oxygen.

On a windy day, continue the experiment. Run some strides with the wind...relax, stretch out and fly along. Then try running into the wind. Lean into it and take shorter strides while using a forceful arm action. Pump your arms a little extra by pushing them backwards, allowing them to come forward to their natural height before forcing them rapidly back again.

Lower arms go forward and back, not across the chest. Keep the elbows close to your side, flexed at 90 degrees. Keep your shoulders directly above the hips to prevent trunk rotation; don't hunch forward or pull your shoulders back. Keep your head nicely balanced above your hips too.

When running into the wind, keep the knees low. This reduces your stride length, so that you're in the air for less time on each stride. The less time in the air, the less it has a chance to push you back. Make the calves propel you forward...not upwards. A half-inch too high in the air can cost you 10 percent of your energy, so decrease your vertical bounce and run forwards instead of up.

Artificial surfaces and football fields are useful for speed running. Be aware of the slope or camber though. Running across a severe slope is bad for the ankles, knees and hips; run up over the center of the field from the sidelines.

A good way to run fast is from corner to corner across the field. This will give you about 130 meters. To recover, jog the side of the field. As you get fitter, you can jog the end of the playing area, which is about 30 to 40 meters shorter than the length. This session is particularly good in the depths of winter when many paths are too muddy for fast running. However, don't deny yourself resistance sessions by avoiding the mud!

Lung capacity also increases with speed training. A 5 foot 10 inch, 20 year-old male has a 3,200 cc lung capacity at age 20. By the age of 50 he has lost 350 ccs of that capacity. Breathing deeply many times each week improves your diaphragm...which is the main weapon of breathing. The auxiliary breathing muscles, the muscles of the abdomen, chest, including the intercostals, are also developing more strength and endurance. You'll gradually regain vital lung capacity, or maintain most of your capacity if you exercise as you age. As a result, you'll find steady runs easier. Breathing in takes muscle action; expiration is mostly passive, the result of muscles relaxing. You forcefully exhale too though, but don't waste much effort.

Once or twice a day, practice breathing deeper than you normally would. Sense your interior stretch receptors sending messages as you fully expand your chest...taking in pint after pint of air. Adopt a good upright posture for this exercise. Do these exercises to ensure you get the maximum capacity genetics has allowed you. Train your lungs. You can also look up "respiratory inhalation resistance trainers" or similar on the internet to find this weeks $20 to $30 deep breathing trainers.

Let pleasant thoughts pass through your mind when you do these breathing exercises: the lovely wife you will be seeing later; the trees and flowers on your next run; your running style compared to a faster runner; choosing the one TV show to watch before or after one of your other hobbies this evening. Build up those intercostal muscles just like you are building your leg muscles: they are all running muscles.

Organelles called mitochondria are the energy factories within cells, which give your muscles zip. They take fuel (sugar usually, though in the form of ATP) and another fuel (oxygen) and...with the nerve to ignite...wham...you get the punch to drive your bones and joints down the trail. The steady runs and gentle speed stuff has increased the number and size of your mitochondria, and increased the capillaries to bring in these fuels. Your muscle fibers have also grown in size, and they can contract more times per minute...you have more endurance and more power.

Running faster requires slight adjustments to the format of training sessions. All speed sessions from Chapter 5 to 11 need a warmup of ten to fifteen minutes of steady running, followed by the stretches from Chapter Three. This warmup procedure prepares your muscles for working hard. Muscles are more efficient when warm and are less likely to strain. Speed running can then be done with minimal injury risk.

After the speed element do five to ten minutes of steady running. Take care with your cooldown. Don't come to a sudden stop because fast running leaves harsh chemicals in your system. Get into the habit of doing easy running after all speed sessions. Then repeat the gentle stretching. The more blood you can move through your exercised muscles after a session the quicker they recover. Sore muscles need rest too. A walk, a warm bath or shower may also help.

Really achy afterwards? Cooler showers, a cool bath, followed by ice applications help. Or walk into cold water up to your waist soon after your run. 65 degrees F is preferable, but 85 F is cool enough to get rid of muscle heat and to decrease inflammation.

As your legspeed increases, you will feel more relaxed on steady runs and enjoy your running much more.

Find the speed which feels natural to you and you're less likely to hurt yourself. Find a comfortable stride rate and stride length, and then as you work on one aspect of your form at a time, your entire running form will become smoother. Think about being graceful.

Fast running will improve your flexibility. Power yourself forward with the calves to extend your stride.

Land close to a point under your center of gravity, with a flexed knee, to prevent pounding or jarring. Float as if running across hot coals, but don't tense up in anticipation of landing on hot coals.

You may want to strip down to shorts for this faster running, although on chilly days, you should feel relaxed with a track suit bottom or sweats on. The main consideration will be the conditions. Having raised the body temperature slightly in the warmup, you must maintain it. In winter, or on windy days all through the year, this can require two or more layers on your top half, and a light covering on the legs to keep the chill off.

If the temperature is below about 40 degrees, or warmer but windy, the cold becomes a potential danger. Treat cold with respect...collapsing when training hard in winter is not uncommon. Plan ahead. To prevent the body from cooling down on very cold or windy days your recovery should be short.

Fartlek Running.

After a few sessions of 100s you can move onto fartlek training. A park or forest with dirt trails is the ideal venue. After warming up, run round the park or trails at an easy pace with striders of 50 to 200 meters at modest pace as and when you feel like it. Run easy or walk between efforts. Stride up some small hills, and ease effortlessly down others. This is speedplay and is of most use when feeling run-down or tired. Just put on your running gear and go; get in touch with your inner child...to keep running fun.

Don't run so fast that your breathing becomes labored. Run slow enough that you can run a dozen pick-ups of 100 meters or more. Fartlek tips:

* Run on soft surfaces such as grass or dirt.
* Pick a tree or lamppost and stride toward it.
* Or, use your watch timer to run moderately fast for 30 to 60 seconds, recover at easy pace for the same amount of time.
* Stride up a few gentle hills.
⁺ Go to a track, run the straights, and jog the curves.
* While running anywhere, count the number of footfalls. Run fairly fast for 30 to 40 foot strikes with the left foot; run easy to recover and repeat several times.
* Run no faster than 90 percent of your maximum heartrate until you have done 10 sessions and also until you've reached 10 minutes at speed. You can then increase your intensity to reach 95 percent of your max HR toward the end of speed sections, which should be your 5K race pace.

Trail Running

When the surface is uneven, your muscles compensate to keep you balanced; rough ground will make you work harder to achieve the same speed. Early trail sessions can be shorter because you'll be putting in more effort per minute. Let the ankles roll with the terrain, building up the small muscles of the lower legs. Later, increase the duration of your run to 40 minutes on this surface. See "Trail finder" at www.trails.com for thousands of places to run.

Adaptations to Speed Training in conjunction with 40 minute runs Include:

* Increased maximum oxygen uptake;
* Increased running efficiency: you stay low to the ground with minimal bouncing and run in straighter lines;
* Flexibility, strength, and coordination improve with aerobic speed running;
* Increased muscle metabolism of fatty acids, which conserves your glycogen or sugar;
* Increased muscle and connective tissue strength;
* Increased fast twitch muscle use: they look and behave more like slow twitch fibers.
* Diaphragm and rib cage muscles improve...therefore;
* Move more air, making more oxygen available;
* More red blood cells (RBCs) are produced;
* More Myoglobin inside your cells, which carries oxygen to the mitochondria;
* More and bigger mitochondria in your muscle cells;
* Blood volume increases...giving the Carbon Dioxide waste a greater reservoir to be excreted in. (Red blood cells bring most of the Oxygen in; the blood plasma or liquid takes two-thirds of the Carbon Dioxide out).
* Stronger heart with a lower resting heart rate decreases the effort needed for a given speed;
* The "other running muscles" get stronger;
* You can run faster before forming excessive lactic acid;

Or to put it another way...Your *Endurance* increases...that is, the ability of your muscle fibers to contract repeatedly at a sub-maximal workload for a prolonged period.

Chapter Six

TWO HUNDREDS

Timed fast running.

After several weeks of 100s and fartlek, you should be ready for some formal speedwork with timed efforts over a set distance. Find somewhere you can run without interruption for about 200 meters. One side of a small sports ground or a section of good forest path will be fine. After the usual warm up and a few relaxed striders of fifty to one hundred meters you can start the 200s.

Stride as you did previously for the 100s. Walk back as a recovery and repeat the 200. This time, run a little faster. Don't commence a strider if your pulse is above 120 per minute at the end of the recovery. Time each one. When the times are increasing, you've had enough. Pace yourself to do ten efforts and don't go above 95 percent of your max HR. They should not be sprints because you will be lucky to manage two of these.

When you feel tired, think about your rhythm...Run smoothly. Cut out exaggerated, unneeded motions.

When your body has got used to this session you can gradually increase the speed. Try running the first few repeats in the same time as (say) the third fastest from the previous session. You should still not be sprinting. When you get fitter, you can take your pulse higher than the earlier guideline, up to 98 percent of your maximum heartrate, which is usually 10 to 15 seconds per mile faster than 5K pace.

Running Form

Running with a moderately high knee lift enables the lower leg to swing through under the knee much faster to start its next stride. The higher the knee lift, the faster the lower leg will swing through, and the longer the stride.

Your knee lift will be lower at longer distances, but a respectable knee lift will help. Take care to avoid overstriding; aches or injuries to the shins and the muscles at the back of the upper legs (hamstrings and gluteals) are one indication of overstriding. These injuries are caused by early fatigue and loss of muscle efficiency.

o   Improving hip flexibility may help
o   Check your form in the last quarter of a training session or race and shorten your stride if you need to.
o   Curb your enthusiasm. Start all runs at a gentle shuffle, lifting the feet just enough to prevent yourself from tripping up. Do the same for the last few minutes of each run. That is, warm up and cooldown for each run.

One oddity of running is that even though the body is moving forward, when your foot touches the ground, the foot should actually be moving backwards. You should then pull the foot back as if grasping a rope (which your ancestors could easily do), and push off from between the first and second toe.

In overstriding, the foot is still traveling forward as it strikes the ground. You may hear a slapping as your feet whack into the ground. The heel then acts as a break, causing stress and damage on every stride. This would be the 'pounding' which other writers' claim runners suffer from. Float along nicely while kissing the ground to avoid muscle and joint damage; flow across the terrain by finding the stride length that suits you. Your stride length will possibly increase as you become stronger, and then decrease again as you find its natural length.

Find a nice running groove while looking about 50 meters ahead of you for the most part, which keeps your head in the right spot. However, look even farther ahead for future impediments like turns, mud or traffic, and note the area just a few yards ahead when you're approaching uneven terrain or curbs. If you spend your running life looking at your feet all the time, you'll miss almost everything…except the obstacle coming toward you, the curb, or a car!

One way to avoid overstriding is to run at high cadence, which means at fast legspeed. You'll have to take shorter strides, yet you cover more ground per minute...exactly what you've been practicing for the last few weeks.

Once you've improved your legspeed, you can make the session help your endurance. Endurance is improved by reducing the recovery period. Instead of walking back, jog slowly. A second option is to jog away briefly at the end of each 200 meter strider, then turn around to jog back to where you finished: then run (and time) another strider the other way. Aim to run the second of each pair at the same speed as the first one.

Keep good leg cadence while you're working on your endurance with this session; don't allow your legspeed to decrease.

In the early sessions of 200s, check your pulse a few times at the end of the recovery. If it's not down to 120 per minute, you should slow your running speed or increase the rest period. The heart recovers about 60 percent of its composure within one minute, so take short rests.

Your training schedule should now look like this:
Repeat the two weeks several times for up to three months.

Sat – 40 mins including 20 mins fartlek in woods
Sun – 40 mins steady run at 65 % max heartrate
Mon – warmup, 10 x 200 meters with a 200 slow jog recovery; get
          up to 95 percent of your maximum heartrate.
Tues – gentle cross training each week
Wed – 40 mins including a few small hills
Thur – 40 mins at 75 percent of max heartrate
Fri – rest each week

Sat – Fartlek in a park, striding up and down gentle hills
Sun – 40 min steady
Mon – 35 min steady
Wed – warmup, 20 mins of 100 meter striders on grass alternating
          with easy running to work on relaxed high knee lift action.
Thur – 40 min at 75 percent max heartrate

Fast running does put additional stress on the body. You develop strong running muscles or agonists, but you may create an imbalance in the antagonistic muscles, which complement the work of running muscles.

The calf muscles work very hard in several phases of the stride, especially push off, or toe off: The calves become very strong. The calf is the agonist or prime mover. The calf muscles complementary muscle at the front of the shin is relatively weak. The Tibialis Anterior...the muscle in front of and to the side of the Tibia bone of the lower leg doesn't work against the ground. It is mostly a resistor or complementary muscle to the calf.

Once the calf muscles have finished contracting at push off, with the foot (hopefully) at full extension, the calf mus-cles...muscle fiber by muscle fiber...relax. The fibers in the calf muscle gradually return to their resting length. The toes and the rest of the lower foot move back to its neutral position...but not merely by the calf muscles relaxing. The tibialis anterior muscle comes into play. It contracts, speeding the foot back to a neutral position.

The shin muscle is relatively small and weak. Complementary or antagonist muscles are often the first to strain. To avoid this, you should consider the following exercises before and after running: Do each for one minute to decrease injuries to weak areas.

* To strengthen the shin muscles: sit on a table, legs hanging down. Dangle a 5 to 10 pound weight from the toes; lift the toes up to raise the weight. Hold for 10 seconds and repeat four times.
* To decrease knee problems: position as above, raise the leg to the horizontal, hold for ten seconds and repeat four times. Do abductor exercises because the abductors keep the hip and knee stable during the support phase of each stride. Lie on your side and raise the upper leg 10 times for a count of 5. Switch legs and do 2 sets.
* Low back pain: do sit-ups with knees bent and heels close to your buttocks; build to one minute of a steady flowing action. Try sit-backs. Start in the up position, then keeping the back straight, ease your shoulders toward the floor. Hold the position about halfway down, and then go back up. Keep your neck straight and relaxed with your hands at, but not pulling on your ears.
* Hamstrings: lie face down; curl the lower leg to touch the buttock. Or, sit on a wheeled office chair and walk your way around the office or up the corridor to exercise the muscles at the back of your legs!

* <u>Glutei or gluteals:</u> from the kneeling or standing position, push one leg backwards and upwards as high as you can; hold up for ten seconds; repeat four times per leg.

* Before all speed running sessions, do a few leg swings for the sprinting muscles which are used at full extension and full flexion. Stand at right angles to something that you can hold onto for balance. After making sure there is no one and nothing which you will kick at your front or rear, rise up onto the toes of the leg closest to the support, and then swing the outer leg forward and backward through its full range of motion at the hip joint. Do 10 to 12 gentle rhythmic cycles and then turn around to do the other leg.

You may only need one or two of these exercises. Listen to your body. Try to spot your weak points, and then incorporate these exercises into your 30 minute weight training sessions!

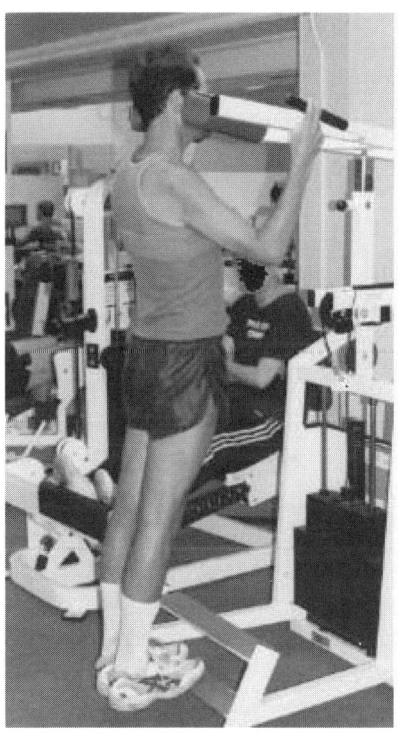

Achilles tendon hurting? Faster running may have given you a tender Achilles due to the heel tab on your shoes digging in on every stride, bruising the Achilles.

<u>Cut off the tabs.</u> Take a few days off from running to let the swelling subside, take NSAIDs for a week, and then do this pictured stretch.

Then strengthen the muscles with calf raises. Stand on a step and raise yourself up on your toes. Allow the heels to drop slowly down below step height, and then push up rhythmically. Then ease back into running.

Note that he is not weight training by pushing weights up with his calves; his shoulders are well below the bar. He <u>is</u> maintaining a light grip on the handle with two fingers to pull himself up if he feels too much strain on the calf muscles while stretching.

Do one set of weights and you'll get 75 percent of the benefits of three sets. Do one set of weights, three days a week and you get 225 percent of the training benefit of doing three sets of weights in one session! You do not need excruciatingly long, hard sessions in the weight room. Do 12 repeats on 12 to 15 different exercises to cover most of the body. Want one all inclusive exercise? Dream on. However, the leg-press, or if you have no equipment, the half squat or lunge all exercise most of the big running muscles.

MORE ON RUNNING FORM

Consider these running form tips and check Chapter Eleven.

Run upright or perpendicular to the ground. Don't lean forward up hills. Don't run as if you're about to sit down...with your weight behind you. Run tall and proud.

Some people need to pull their shoulders back.

Bring the hips forward to move the center of gravity over the midfoot, which is where you should land on each stride.

Make your foot hug your buns on the swing-through.

On every stride, lift your heel close to your buns. This will give you a faster stride rate. One way to practice this is with bun flicks. Run along for twenty seconds and flick your feet rapidly up to touch your bottom. Take very short strides forward because moving up the track or field is not the main purpose. Some people call this exercise high heels because you flick the heels up to your buttocks. Others call them butt kicks.

A second drill is to practice very short, but fast stride while flicking yourself forward using the calf muscles. This conditions the calves and improves legspeed.

Next, use the quadriceps and the Ilio-soas muscles (hip flexors) at the front of the leg, to whip the leg through. To prepare for this, practice high knee raises while running on the spot or moving a few inches at a time up the track. Practice a high knee skipping action too. Bring in rapid arm movements to increase your leg speed. After three or four 15 second efforts at this, practice running at moderate pace while whipping the leg through. Your knees don't need to be high like a sprinter. Leg speed is the key.

Practice these three drills separately, then together as you hug the buns with your foot AND pull the leg through fast.

Don't run with your face. Relax the facial muscles and let your jaw drop, otherwise you'll transfer the tension to the rest of your body.

Most of the muscles for running set up the calf muscles to propel you forward. A good push off from the toes is best achieved by extending the trail leg while pushing off from the end of the toes. You'll need to maintain good ankle flexibility to do this, and then pull your leg through fast for the next stride.

Move your arms smoothly; feel in control. Arms help your legs to know where they are in the stride cycle. Don't allow the arms to go very high in the front; go just high enough to stop the shoulders from rolling.

Keeping the arms smooth will also decrease your head roll. Head movement is rarely a good thing. Head rolling in speedwork or racing is a waste of energy and will slow you down. Keep your neck and shoulders relaxed. You rarely see world record holders with head movement. The eyes should not wander much either, except to take in the periphery. Keep your eyes focused about 50 meters ahead of you. Don't lift your shoulders up when you pick up speed. Keep them low and relaxed.

Keep your elbows bent at about 90 degrees. Don't actively lock the elbows in place, but keep them at roughly the right angle...stable yet loose. Avoid bringing the lower arms across the body...the arms need to go straight back and straight forward just like your legs do. Your legs should not kick off to the side either.

Relax your hands...stay loose as if softly holding onto an egg.

Use a natural style. Think of being at ease...at play. Let the feet roll you down the path. Stride smoothly.

Land with a slightly flexed knee but don't lock the knee.

Don't land daintily on the toes. Do land softly on the outer midfoot or outer heel. Then roll inwards a bit and off the toes.

While knee lift is important, don't copy sprinters.

But don't shuffle along either. Hug the ground as you propel yourself forward in the horizontal plane...not the vertical.

Don't waste energy with long strides. Too long a stride makes you lose momentum. Taking strides a few inches shorter can help you to run faster. The quadriceps want to devour the ground...let them, but keep them in check.

Find your ideal stride length: it will change according to your running speed.

Practice making your feet go straight forward, rather than throwing your feet to the side on each stride, which makes the hip swivel. Practice running in a straight line. Run straight for less waste and more speed.

Let the tension out of your muscles as your finely trained machine cruises in harmony to the end of the block, track or to the next tree. Stay light on your feet until you ease to a jog for 30 to 60 seconds rest.

Going getting tough such as when running up a hill? Maintain realistic pace in an upright position and imagine being pulled up to the sky. Wind a bit stiff? You're a sleek mach two aircraft slicing through the air. Studly horses cantering away from you at the one-mile point in a 5K? Many can only gallop for a mile; you can lope along strongly for days.

Think about one aspect of your form for a few minutes on every run. An efficient running style will save you energy and decrease your potential for injury. The more practice you have, the more efficient you will become. You will get faster.

Some people run a little differently because of their body shape, their biomechanics. If readers feel awkward using the above style, they should use what feels natural to them. A leg length operation or orthotics may cure them, of course. If you want to improve, seek out experts to check for leg length differences.

An orthotic will enable some people to run with more efficiency...with less effort. You should all aspire to run fast with minimal effort.

Stop the speed session for a minute when your form deteriorates. Gather your mental energy and do four more gentle striders to practice good form with tired muscles. This will help you maintain good form at the end of a 5K race.

If you've raced at the 5K, your speed running can be up to 10 seconds per mile faster than race pace, but you still do not need to sprint and injure yourself. Stay in control at modest speed. Although those four extra striders are worthwhile, don't discourage yourself by doing long, hard speed sessions.

If you're not careful, the harsh ground contact of fast running tenderizes your muscles, so don't overstride. Speed running will strengthen the muscles and connective tissue, but bones take several months to reach peak strength: they can also take three months to mend. Don't over stress your bones and ligaments early on, or you'll take 13 weeks off of running with a fracture. Bones take months to gain the full physiological strength from training.

Use your mouth to breathe because the orifice is bigger,

and you don't have to worry about it being stuffed up. The length of tubing (dead space) is less. Forget the 'in-the-nose...out-the-mouth routine.' You don't have to concentrate on it if you mouth breathe. Take rhythmic long deep breaths because 150 cc of tidal breath is dead space, a section of air which goes in and out with each breath, yet is not replaced. You don't wear a mouthguard, so you don't need tape on your nose to breathe right!

Actually, while mouth breathing you're taking in about one-third of your air via the nose. The negative pressure in the lungs simply pulls in air via mouth and nose even if it feels like it's only the mouth that lets air in.

Relaxation at Speed.

There is more to speed and fast races than powering down the road or track. You also need to relax. Run at 90 percent effort and 10 percent relaxation for better performance. At 100 percent physical effort, your muscles tense up, wasting precious energy. As you read a few pages back, muscles work in pairs. The hamstrings must relax while the quadriceps are contracting or else they are fighting each other, and tighten up. Relaxing helps you to run smoother or economically, thus increasing your speed at maximum oxygen use (or your velocity at maximum VO2), which gives you faster races.

Relax before and during running to:

* Increase blood flow to the muscles, reduce cramps and make the motion more fluid. Which:
* Decreases the formation of lactic acid. And:
* Reduces fatigue because of less tension in your muscles.
* Practice relaxation with deep breathing exercises, a few yoga positions, meditation, biofeedback, music or gentle running and stretching prior to speed running.

Practice the deep breathing exercises of page 65 to encourage slow breathing. While at rest, inhale slowly, pushing the abdomen in to fill up the thorax and the lower part of your lungs. Then draw your shoulders back to ensure the upper part of the lungs fully inflate. Hold for 3 to 5 seconds, and then exhale slowly. After a couple of seconds with nearly empty lungs, repeat the inhalation. British researchers have shown that endurance improves with forceful breathing exercises.

Practice belly breathing while supine. Place your hand or a book on your belly, and make sure that the belly goes up and down while you breathe. The chest should barely move up as the lungs inflate. As you take 17 to 23 thousand breaths per day, you may as well get it right. As mentioned before, mouth breathe during exercise.

The Shuffle Option.

Beware of too high a knee lift. You may run faster by keeping your feet closer to the ground. High knee lift will waste energy...you go vertical instead of horizontal.

The shuffle is a ground hugging style and is more economical for many people. You still push off from the toes properly, but you keep your feet close to the ground in all phases of the stride, saving energy with less vertical bounce. Yes...the stride length will shorten, but leg speed can be increased to compensate.

Practice raising those feet so they barely slither above the surface...No forward lean. Run tall with rapid strides. As you set off, think short rapid strides and feel your cadence change. When on trails, pick your feet up a bit to avoid branches and rocks.

The key to gaining fitness is to build up your body rather than wearing it down. Rest days allow your body systems to repair and get stronger. You can also alternate harsh runs with easier runs to get the same hard-easy method of training used by Olympians.

After several months of 200s and fartlek, you might wish to take your Interval training to higher levels. You'll run at 5K pace to 2-mile race pace, using repeats of 300 to 800 meters. But not yet. Cruise through Chapters 7 to 9, and after you've raced a few 5Ks, see Chapter 10 and 11 for higher intensity training.

Chapter Seven

LONG REPETITIONS

Racing requires a constant fast pace. So far, you've developed endurance with steady running, and some speed and endurance with short strides. Now you will combine them as a prelude to running and eventually racing a few 5Ks.

As you've read elsewhere in this book, most of your runs are not workouts per se, and you should not feel as if they are training. However, you have practiced running for 40 minutes continuously and you have practiced the art of running respectably fast. Because you've made such subtle changes to the length of your runs and to how fast you do your striders, no <u>one</u> particular session should feel like training. However, the four or five runs per week represent a training program, and the combination of sessions is getting you fitter.

Despite the fact that you are only running at 60 to 75 percent of maximum heartrate most of the time, you'll have a few sections which feel harsh. Some days you'll also feel fatigue. Osteoblasts are busy depositing a matrix, which is calcifying by the day and making your bones stronger. Osteoclasts are shaping this new bone. Don't rush into still harder training.

This chapter gives you another chance to play the game of running, and you'll take your muscles to a modest level of fatigue for several minutes at a time. You will do your usual warmup and stretches before doing these sessions.

The striders that you've been doing are fun and developed your leg speed. You need to get the quadriceps used to coming up higher, and to using your hamstrings and butt muscles properly by running upright but not uptight. Pushing off from the end of the toes also saves the quads energy.

So far, you've been running at speeds which enable you to provide all the oxygen requirements of your body as you run. In so-called aerobic running, the muscles work with sufficient oxygen. The striders are so short that you don't get into oxygen debt either.

However, when you run fast for long periods, the oxygen system will not be able to keep up, and the anaerobic pathway will break down part of your ATP or sugar.

The aerobic system will provide as much energy as it can; only the deficit will be made up by the anaerobic system. Both systems operate at all times, but the anaerobic system becomes more important for sudden intense efforts, such as running up hills. In a race, the anaerobic system supplements the aerobic system; it only provides a few percent of your total energy needs.

There is a cost to anaerobic running: You produce lactic acid, which accumulates in the muscles and contributes slightly to your feeling of fatigue, encouraging you to slow down.

To delay this anaerobic poisoning of the muscles, you developed your heart and lungs with steady running...then further stimulated them with the strides over short distances at a moderate effort. These two forms of running have developed your aerobic system to good effect but it will be years before you reach your maximum potential.

Now you can improve your ability to run anaerobically...by introducing sessions which create a slight build up of lactic acid. The acid is not dangerous, it is merely a natural, though slowing by-product of fast running.

The first stage is to run moderately fast for three to four minutes...and do so several times within a training session. The recovery between efforts will be a walk at first.

When you're used to the session, you can jog during the recovery. For the first few sessions, the walking or jogging should last as long as the fast part. Later you can reduce the rest period toward one minute.

As discussed in Chapter 6, running fast creates extra stresses on the body. It's not only the muscles that feel the strain...joints, tendons and ligaments experience additional work.

You can lesson the strain on these parts by aiming to run re-laxed...in control. Just like with the 200s of Chapter Six, land soft rather than pounding. Decrease your stride length to land softer, as if onto egg shells. Form is especially vital during the last minutes of each repetition because you're more likely to develop poor mechanics when tired. So, run within your own body limits. Reduce injury risk by holding back during the first two minutes.

Run on soft surfaces such as packed dirt or sand, grass, or synthetic tracks. Fairly smooth trails are excellent for these long sections of fast running; easing through bends or nasty footing for a few seconds and then picking up the pace will not spoil the affects of the session. Or use the edge of a large recreation ground. Run two-thirds of it fast and use the other third as the recovery. You could use the length of a favorite piece of road, but avoid con-crete because it's six to ten times harder than asphalt.

It helps to use permanent start and finish points to assist your timing. Timing repeats make it easier to monitor your progress. A large tree or the corner of a building are effective points to use.

Your first session of long reps.

After warming up for at least a mile, do your usual stretching. Run a few relaxed 50 to 100 meter strides. Then start your three minute repetition. Don't run too fast, but you should be feeling quite tired by the end. If you've raced before at the 5K, your pace should be about 25 to 35 seconds per mile slower than 5K pace. Although you'll be running slower than in the last chapter, your pulse will go up to 80 to 85 percent of your maximum. It should soon return to 120. Once it's done so, you're ready to go again.

Do the second repetition and think more about your running style. Try to keep a steady rhythm going...especially for the second half. Let the tension go from the shoulders, maybe drop the arms a little, but keep them moving fast and allow your legs to carry you through.

The leg muscles should feel a little heavy with the fatigue of anaerobic running, but after an active rest, you should persevere with the third repetition.

This time, start a little slower. As you reach halfway, pick your knees up to extend or to speed up your stride. Don't extend it so much, and go so fast, that you collapse on the ground afterwards. Complete the session with a significant amount to spare. Feel as if you could run another rep, but do your warmdown instead. The real work will come in later sessions, when you aim to improve your times by a few seconds toward 10K pace or about 20 seconds per mile slower than 5K pace. You will also reduce the rest period by jogging a bit faster between repeats.

When you've done Chapter 11s Intervals, you can run long repeats at or a little faster than 5K pace. But that's many months away, so for now, enjoy yourself at 30 seconds per mile slower than 5K pace.

The first time you do this session should be after a rest day. If you're very stiff afterwards, you've overdone it. Any new type of training is hard to judge at first. Running the repeats on a 400 meter track will help you to judge the pace. If you think you were too fast on the first repetition, consider stopping for the day. You could run half a dozen short striders to unwind.

A week later you can repeat the session and judge the pace better. As with your 200s in Chapter Six, aim for your times to get faster during a session. Do not run a fastest time by ten seconds for the first repeat, and follow it with slow efforts.

After doing the above session twice, you should find a second area to run fast for five to six minutes.

Run two efforts of this five to six minute route or loop. Run the first half at 5 to 10 seconds per mile slower than the speed of your three minute route...then speed up by those 5 to 10 seconds per mile for the extra two minutes. You'll need about 5 minutes recovery, so jog or walk to stay warm for the second effort.

You will eventually run the entire 6 minute repeat at the same pace you currently do for your three minute area, and reduce the recovery to two minutes or less. When you're ready for more stimulation, you can try a 9 to 10 minute loop.

You'll need to focus on the right pace for the first few minutes, then focus on relaxed effort to maintain pace.

Only run long repeats once a week. Alternating the area and the length of the repetitions will give you variety.

It's far better to go faster by two or three seconds per repetition than to go slower for each one as the session progresses. Going faster makes you feel in control.

Going slower for consecutive reps makes you feel un-comfortable...demoralizing you for future sessions of this type. You'll dread the sessions; soon you'll avoid this type of training. You're likely to experience some sessions in which you slow, but use your will-power to curtail your speed in the first few minutes to keep errors to a minimum.

To race fast you must train fast, but this fast running must feel relaxed. Maintain your form to be economical, just like you did in prior Chapters. Try to gain a sense of relaxation at speed...at what is quite close to race pace.

Every time you do this session, you further train your muscle fibers for operating in the presence of lactic acid. You increase your lactate buffering capacity. You push back your anaerobic threshold. You'll also learn to run more efficiently at this intensity, add to the number and size of your mitochondria, increase healthy enzyme activity, produce more Myoglobin and even more capillaries. Your endurance will improve. The seven-minute miles, which were at your threshold pace a few weeks ago, will soon feel easy; you'll soon run 6:55 miles at threshold pace.

Some people say soreness after these sessions is due to lactic acid remaining in the muscles, but the soreness is mostly from basic fatigue and a few microscopic muscle fiber tears...which will heal and result in stronger muscles if given sufficient rest. You could lay on the grass for half an hour after the last rep (something you might be tempted to do if you've run them too fast), and nearly all the lactic acid would be gone...absorbed by your system. However, it's still better to do a cooldown to bring a steady supply of blood to the muscles, and to get rid of lingering pockets of lactic acid. While a mile of running is probably best to unwind, walking is fine if you're too pooped to run easy, though it probably means that you ran too fast during your repeats. Comfortably harsh is the correct intensity, or about 85 percent of maximum heartrate. Not up to running after the session? Any gentle activity will reduce the potential for stiffness.

As you learn how to pace yourself, and to run more economically, the times for these weekly reps will decrease substantially. The next level of improvement will come after your buffering system has adapted: the decrease in your times may not be as profound. Restrain yourself from racing these repeats...and move onto the next chapter.

Your **basic training schedule** is much like the last chapter, but you can run your long repeats each Saturday.

Saturdays – Use a three week rotation of:
    3 to 4 minute repeats or half-mile efforts.
    5 to 6 minute repeats or 1,200 meter efforts.
    9 to 10 minute repeats or mile efforts.
Sun – 40 min steady
Mon – fartlek in a park, striding up and down gentle hills
Tues – rest
Wed – warmup, 10 mins of 100 meter striders on grass (e.g. 30 seconds fast, then 30 seconds easy or walking) work on relaxed high knee lift action. Then 10 mins of 200 meter striders (or 60 seconds fast alternating with 60 seconds slow). Or do 20 to 30 x 100 meters one week and 10 to 16 x 200s the next week.
Thur – 40 min at 75 percent max heartrate
Fri – rest

You would also be doing some cross training each week.

According to the Journal of Medical Science for Sport & Exercise, speed at lactate threshold is the best physiologic predictor of endurance event performance. Your oxygen use at lactate threshold or LTVO2 is also talked about by physiologists, but as you're unlikely to measure it, we'll stick with threshold pace. You can increase your speed at threshold pace by stimulating or stressing your current threshold many times each week using repetitions.

Stimulate your anaerobic threshold by running at or slightly faster than threshold. Run 10 percent of your weekly miles at 15 to 25 seconds slower than 10K pace, or 27 to 37 seconds per mile slower than 5K pace. Run a series of efforts from half a mile to two miles with only a one minute rest between efforts. See also the speed table and notes in Chapter 15 to help you decide on the appropriate pace to run.

Peace and quiet for fast running.

Choose a time of day when your repetition area has fewest distractions for you. Avoid:

- Popular dog walking times;
- School chuck-out time;
- Busy trails at the weekend.

It's easy to cope with people in a park when you're doing striders because it makes little difference which part of a field you use, or whether it's 100 or 150 meters; you can change the distance according to the area available that day.

You need tranquillity when running long repeats. Don't let other people add to your running stress. Running is supposed to decrease life's stress, not add to it. Notice how you feel, not just what your watch tells you. When conditions are bad, 4:10 can be worth your sub 4 minute repetition when everything is perfect.

You can run one in four of the long rep sessions on a 400 meter synthetic or dirt track from the very beginning of this Chapter. Half-miles and mile repeats are the most logical. The main advantage is that wherever you are in the country, give or take two meters (440 yards or a quarter mile is about 402 meters), most tracks are the same size. Track repeats will improve your pace judgment because you can check lap splits on each repeat. Note: Run two laps in lane 6 and you'll get 867 meters; 4 laps will be 1734 meters and decrease your leaning and injury risk.

In later months or years, your long repeats will be close to 5K pace; a smooth surface is a great tool for achieving 5K pace. Your tempo runs of the next chapter will be 25 to 35 seconds per mile slower than 5K pace, so road, trail, grass or a flat beach with firm sand are better training areas.

Remember to do your 4 striders before the long repeats. Although your goal is to practice running with a little lactic acid in your blood and muscles, a proper warmup, including striders before speed running means that you will produce less lactic acid during your long repeats. A study in Medicine & Science in Sports & Exercise found the same holds true for cyclists, so when you cross train, do your warmup and a few 15 second efforts before the serious speed cycling.

Chapter Eight

TEMPO RUNS

After doing long repetition sessions for at least six weeks, you should be ready to bring in a weekly sustained run. Kudos to the author for giving you a three week rotation of Saturday repeats. Go through those twice, then rest up by 25 percent for a race at the end of the seventh week; a 5K would be ideal.

Sustained running is fast running, sustained over a longish period of time. Another name for it is Tempo running because you maintain a fast continuous tempo. The initial target is to run for 15, building to 20 minutes. The pace will be faster than your steady runs, but can be a few seconds per mile slower than your long repetitions.

You will run at 80 to 90 percent of your maximum heartrate. As in the last chapter, you'll push back the lactate or anaerobic threshold. Cruise moderately hard on these runs. Focus on your form...including your toe push off, the amount of knee raise, stride length and correct arm swing.

Heartrate is the key. The pace should feel somewhat harsh but you must feel in control. Weather conditions and how you feel will determine how fast you run on a given day.

One of the problems of Tempo running is overheating. For the last six weeks, you've worked for three to five minutes with a rest to recover. If you walk around in a shaded area on hot days, this also lets your body dissipate some of its heat. Even at close to freezing point, you may find these Tempo sessions are best done without sweats or tights to allow for additional cooling.

Half of your improvement in lactate threshold or turnpoint is achieved in a mere 3 sessions or less than 2 weeks.

It takes about 12 weeks to get the full benefits, and another 12 weeks before your VO2 max reaches its highest level from these threshold sessions.

Running is about patience. If you increase your weekly mileage by 5 miles next year, it will again take 24 weeks to see the full benefits.

At some point in the 24 weeks, you'll also need to convert 2 of the 5 miles to gentle speed running!

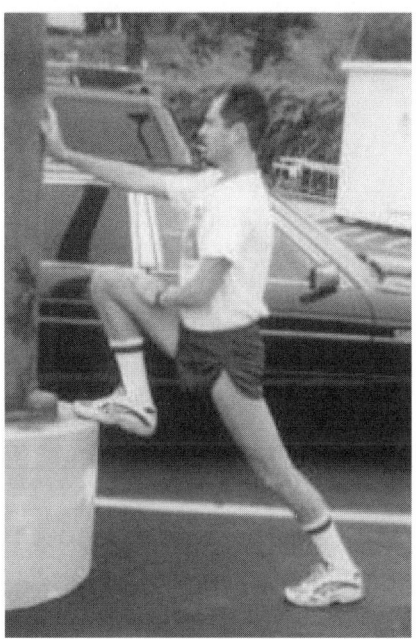

The leg stretch above is great before tempo running because it stretches almost *all of your running muscles in just 60 seconds. Do it after your warm up and switch legs after 30 seconds.*

On really hot days run your tempo sessions a little slower. Or adjust the time of day that you run to take advantage of cooler conditions. On hot days run with the wind on the way out and enjoy the cooling affect of running into the wind on the way back.

For chilly days, it's probably best to have the easy running in the second half of the run. So, run into the wind on the way out, and you'll be pushed back on the return.

As usual, bring in the new training gradually. After a warmup, stretching such as the leg stretch and short strides, take off your excess gear. Start running a set route or loop, perhaps one that would take you 25 minutes at a steady pace. At the beginning, you should run barely faster than 75 % of max heartrate. After five minutes, increase the pace a bit...then increase again at say eight and eleven minutes...but still run slower than during your long repetition speed of the previous few weeks.

Don't push yourself to collapse during tempo runs. Run at a speed where you feel as if you're under a minimal amount of pressure. Enjoy the sensations from your body as it copes with the run. Feel your old ticker gently pounding in the chest, letting you know it can handle the effort. Enjoy the feeling of those muscles working below full power, but at great effort all the same.

As you read earlier, if you can hear your feet hitting the ground, it can mean your form has broken down due to fatigue; ease off for a minute and take shorter strides to correct your form. Whereas on your steady runs you will have two gears in reserve, on these runs you'll have only one in reserve.

Your heartrate should be about 85 percent of your maximum, but because you don't get rest periods, your running pace will be a bit slower than during your long repetitions. After 15 minutes, ease off for the warmdown. In a few sessions, you'll increase to 20 to 25 minutes of tempo running.

This first attempt can be a target for a time trial in due course. First though, try your next sustained run with a different approach. One week after your first tempo run, assess the pace you think you can carry for the entire length of the run. It should take you to about 85 percent of your maximum heartrate. Set out at this pace and maintain pace at 'comfortably hard,' or at moderate intensity.

Mile markers help you judge pace, but unless accurate, they will give a false indication of speed. Don't get too engrossed in the watch. Use it to help judge the pace, not to race against. Most runners end up with two or three favorite loops for their tempo runs, and the halfway point is of more use than mile points. You'll soon get used to the feel of even pace.

Most coaches agree that you'll find this comfortably hard pace instinctively with practice...yet the running speed will vary week by week according to other things in your life. Don't fight the watch. A heartrate monitor is a better guide; ease your running speed or concentrate on relaxing at your current pace if the monitor shows your heartrate is above 85 percent of your maximum.

Improvement of your times is not the main goal. The main goal is to use a good running style and even pace at 85 percent of your max heartrate. You will eventually run a bit faster for each course, and time trials once a month are useful and fun if you rarely race.

Meantime, enjoy fairly rapid running and make most of these runs a joy by not blasting out too fast.

Find three routes and alternate clockwise with counter-clockwise, and you'll run loops a certain way every six weeks.

week one   route 1 -- steady start getting faster
week two   route 2 -- even pace quite fast
week three   route 3 -- steady start getting faster
week four   route 1 -- even pace quite fast
week five   route 2 -- steady start getting faster
week six   route 3 -- even pace quite fast

One of the routes should include a few small hills if possible, while the others can be mainly flat. In a race, you'll have to take hills in your stride, so practice a relaxed economical way of running hills during tempo runs. The purpose of the tempo run is to prepare you for the stresses of a race...by raising your anaerobic threshold.

The PH of muscle effects muscle enzyme activity: running at threshold pace teaches your muscles to buffer the acid. Psychological fatigue is likely to make you stop exercise at this intensity before your muscles fill up with lactate.

Production of ATP (energy) is twice as fast using anaerobic pathways, but it is only one sixteenth as efficient as aerobic sources. On that basis, perhaps you should restrict yourself to 1/16th of your miles at this pace. However, because most of this running also stimulates better aerobic pathways, you can safely do 10 to 15 percent of your training at threshold pace. Keep most of the other mileage at 70 percent max HR, plus or minus 5 percent.

When you are super fit, your pace at threshold pace should be 25 to 35 seconds per mile slower than 5K race pace, or 15 to 20 seconds slower than 10K pace. When you're super fit, your tempo pace will also reach the same speed as your long repetitions of Chapter 7, and for both types of threshold running, you'll be able to go up to 90 percent of your maximum heartrate.

For some of you, Tempo or threshold running will be at a different pace. Anaerobic threshold is the pace you can sustain for close to an hour, which will be:

*   Half-marathon pace for elite runners;
*   15K or 10 mile pace for excellent club runners;

*   10K pace for many recreational runners.

Use the percentage of your maximum HR to determine your threshold training pace. If you've done one, use the running speed of a 50 to 60 minute race for you as your back-up training pace.

When you're training at Lactate Threshold, you're running in slight oxygen debt because you can't get enough oxygen into the blood stream to prevent the formation of lactic acid.

Training Schedule at 18 to 27 miles per week.

This three week schedule can be can adapted for most runners. As usual, warmup, stretching and strides precede fast running.

Just a reminder. Strides or striders are relaxed 100 meter efforts or runs at about 5K race pace to loosen you up for quality running. Your individual strides will still be 3 to 6 feet or so and you'll do 50 to 70 strides or steps with each foot for each strider or effort, which alas, is also called a stride.

Note that this schedule is based on time, not mileage. The 10-minute mile runner will be doing 4 miles on non-speed days, and 3.5 miles on speed days, for about 18 miles per week. The tempo portion should comprise no more than 15 percent of your total miles each month. After a few weeks, the 10 minute milers will need to increase the tempo part toward 30 minutes.

Cruise easily at 7-minute miles? You'll run about 5.5 miles on your easy days, and 5 miles on speed days, to total about 27 miles per week. Any of you can add 5 minutes per week to the Sunday run to give more endurance, but make sure you'll be fresh enough for Monday's fartlek or striders. All of you should cross-train twice a week. The 24 week rule on page 87 includes your physiologic gains, but not all of your running economy improvement at threshold pace. Running economy changes can give you 5 to 10 years of steady improvement.

Week One

Sat – long repetitions; 3 x three mins, building to 5 repeats after 6 months. Note: after three months and after training through Chapter 11, the pace could edge down to 5K pace or the pace of a 12 to 15 minute time trial. It will then be at about 95 percent of your maximum heartrate instead of this months 85 to 90 percent.

Sun – 40 min steady
Mon – 40 mins: with 20 mins fartlek in woods or on dirt
Tues – rest or gentle cross training every Tuesday.
Wed – sustained run at even pace, quite fast. See how long you can think about your form before you lose your concentration. Then be realistic: think about your form for one minute and work on one or two aspects per session.
Thurs – 40 min steady
Fri   – rest (always)

Week Two
Sat   – long repetitions; 2 x five mins, build toward 3 miles worth at 85 to 90 percent of your maximum heartrate.
Sun – 40 min steady
Mon – 100-meter grass area, 20 mins of strides: work on relaxed high knee lift action with a jog back for recovery.
Wed   – sustained run: steady start, getting faster. Should feel moderately hard, but do run smoothly.
Thurs – 40 min steady

Week Three
Sat – 10 x 200 meters, jog back recovery
Sun – 40 min steady
Mon – 30 mins including 15 mins fartlek in woods
Wed – long repetitions 2 only x three mins relaxed
Thurs – 25 mins steady while resting up to race or time trial
        on Saturday

Note the routine...usually long reps Saturday; short stuff Mondays; rest day on Friday; rotating the sessions as shown in earlier chapters. You don't have to think too deeply about what training to do. This schedule covers and stimulates all of your energy systems.

The easing off in the third week will allow your muscles to adapt to the training and freshen up your legs for a race. You should race only when your body is used to the increased training load, perhaps after six weeks of the sustained (tempo) training. This happens to be two full cycles of three weeks.

Chapter Nine

Racing Tips for the 5K:

Although this book is on 5K running for fun and fitness, many of you will race your 5Ks hard. Please don't start your first few races too fast or it will make your races stressful mentally and physically. If you run your first few races just a few seconds per mile faster than usual Tempo runs, you'll have a more positive experience. You can race faster over ensuing months.

At 5 runs per week, you can consider doing any distance from a one mile fun run to a 5K race. Add half a mile every other week to increase your longest run to 8 miles and you should be able to handle a 10K race. You'll also have more endurance for the 5K!

Your local newspaper's sports section should have a list of up-coming races with contact information to allow you to enter a week or two before the race. You can also search the race data at sites like www.runnersworld.com

Search by race location and distance to find entry information. www.active.com also has a search base and allows you to enter online. Most specialist running stores have race flyers and they often have regional magazines covering a radius of several hundred miles.

Once you've entered the race, ensure that you don't over-train in the final days of preparation. Rest is the most important element over the last few days, but it starts about 10 days pre-race. Whereas you've been used to running for 40 minutes on a Thursday, run a mere 30 minutes on the penultimate weeks Thursday. This will leave you fresher than normal on the Saturday before your race weekend.

Then for the final week:
Sat – 10 x 200 meters, jog back recovery
Sun – 35 min steady
Mon – 25 mins including 10 mins of gentle fartlek in woods
Tues – rest
Wed – long repetitions, but do only 2 x three mins relaxed
Thurs – 20 mins steady prior to a race on Saturday
Fri – make a point of staying off your feet more than usual.
No cross-training this week.

Race Day preparation:
The day before the race: check your race clothing; use your most comfortable shorts and singlet; use good shoes, but not brand new shoes. Racing flats or lightweight shoes may interest you in the future, but for now, use the shoes that accompanied you through your repetition and tempo runs. Stay well hydrated today.

Sports bag: Take 4 small safety pins for your race number (it goes on the front of your racing shirt). Though there will probably be enough food to feed the 10,000 after the race, pack an energy bar, banana and a 32 ounce sports drink, plus water to be sure you get some. You'll also need sunglasses, cap, sunscreen (even on cloudy days), timing chip if used by this race (attach to shoes), lube, change of clothing and a towel.

Get up 2 to 3 hours before a morning race to snack, shower and stretch gently with your running gear on. Or,

4 hours pre race: last meal...light and easily digested such as cereals, toast and banana. Try a small but early lunch for an early afternoon race. You can eat your usual low fat, modest protein, and high carb lunch before an evening race. Coffee or tea should not be a problem if you're used to them. They can stimulate a bowel movement, yet they will not dehydrate you. Stay with the familiar. The American College of Sports Medicine recommends a 400 to 500 calorie meal about 3 hours pre-exercise.

2 hours prerace: Drink some tomato juice for its potassium and sodium, which helps to keep your water content up. Watermelon is a lower sodium source of potassium to keep your heart healthy. Drink enough water to keep your urine pale yellow. One-third

strength fruit juices such as apple are a great energy source during the last two hours. You don't have to buy a sports drink.

Find the race site early to ease your parking hassle and to stay relaxed. Check in to collect your race number if necessary. Some races allow you to pick-up your race number the night before the race. Pin the number on the front of your race shirt…which should be the lightest one you own. A light color to reflect the sun and a light fabric to allow your sweat out. Despite the number of people who wear them, race T-shirts are rarely the ideal shirt to wear.

The Internet, the entry form and running friends were good sources for route information over the last week. If you still need info, find a course map and check for hills. Drive around the course if you can. Decide how fast to start. Uphill starts require restraint. After the hill, you can stretch out and overtake many people who pooped out (actually, runners use the term, died) going up the hill. Steep downhills early demand as much respect as uphills because you'll fatigue your quads if you run them too fast.

Note the finish area and the last half a mile of the race ready for a final surge for the finish.

Rest and hydration are always vital, particularly before a key race.

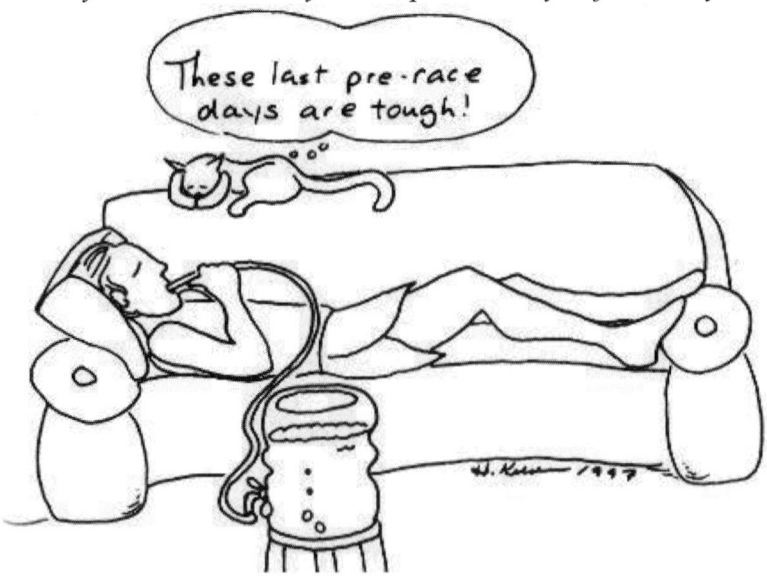

One hour to go: Getting nervous? Tell yourself you're well trained and rested for this race, and that you'll start at a sensible pace and enjoy it. Breathe deeply, relax…it's time for a drink of water if it's hot: if it's not hot...time for a last drink of water. If it's hot...consider the option of a steady start. It's probably time for the bathroom, which may have a long line. Relax, talk and stretch gently while in line. Special trick: Fast food places and service stations within half a mile of the start. Walk/jog there for the bathroom; stretch and then jog back.

Or, 30 minutes to go: ten minutes of easy pace running to warmup. Find somewhere quiet to do your stretching.

15 minutes prerace: put on your race shirt and lighter training shoes if you have them. You will, as always, double-tie your laces. You should not need to take spare laces. If your laces break it implies that the shoes are too old to offer support or that you tie your shoes too tight, which restricts your foot's inner workings.

10 mins prerace: run a few gentle strides near to the start. Not into the wind or up a slope...conserve your energy. Arrange for someone to look after your sweats or exercise tights (if you needed them in the warmup). Hint: At a temperature of 70 or below, it's prudent to keep on a pair of lightweight sweats to maintain muscle warmth while you stretch and relax. Though they are called sweats, you should not be sweating very much. You will strip those sweats off just a few minutes before the start. Your metabolism is now ready for 5K pace running, able to take in lots of oxygen to fuel your warm, injury resistant muscles. Don't start at mile race pace!

If time targets are up, go to a realistic target based on slightly faster than the pace of your sustained runs, or at your current personal record. No time targets on display? Start near the back.

Avoid starting off too fast. The adrenaline flowing makes this hard at times, but the rewards are high if you can achieve it. Your legs soon get tired and also fill up with the wastes of anaerobic running, which results in a labored running action. It is much better to run at an even pace, though the first and last mile are likely to be faster than the middle section.

Negative splits are even better, which means running the second half of the race faster than the first half. This requires restraint for the first mile, something you were practicing in your tempo runs.

Don't take too much notice of your mile or kilometer times, or splits. Even if the entire course is accurate, many of the intermediate mile signs are wrong. Markers have been put out the morning of the race, based on a car's odometer, or attached to the lamppost nearest the actual point, or obliterated.

Used as a guide, mile markers are useful; within a hundred meters, most are correct. In a 10K race, the two or three mile, or 5K point may be the most benefit to you. If you can think straight, average your mile times to give yourself a more accurate picture. Arithmetically challenged? Write your mile split times on a piece of tape or bandaid and place it on your wrist.

Running at even effort is vital. Your easy week will make your legs feel fresh. The Wednesday speed session was to practice pace judgment with fresh legs. On race day, don't run faster than you planned for just because you feel nifty and fresh in the first half a mile. Steady is the key. If you can keep your heartrate within 10 beats per minute of your average for the race, you'll race better. A surge at each mile point may make you feel good while you're doing it, but it will cost you before the race is over.

The faster you start, the more likely you are to hurt early in the race. In fact, don't look for any pain in the first few races. Enjoy the day and achieve times which you'll beat later...while perhaps hurting a bit as you reach your full race potential.

Warmdown after the race. Race recovery starts with 10 minutes of walking or easy running to cooldown from the race, plus liquid and a snack of mostly carbo and a bit of protein to keep your muscles happy (to help them recover).

You'll have to distinguish between physical and mental fatigue in your early races. Picture yourself crossing the finish line with good running form and a smile.

Practice will help you cope with any self-inflicted stresses. Run the first few races with minimal time or place targets and you will not have an Olympians jitters. In a couple of years you can get really nervous at your Olympics when you try for your first sub 30 or sub 20 minute 5K. On those days, just like in your early races, fatigue is likely to be from:

* Dehydration: Start your 5K one percent dehydrated and you add 3 percent to your time: your 24:59 5K becomes 25:44;
* Lack of carbohydrate: Atkins, South Beach and Low Carb eaters beware;
* Starting the race too fast: A steady, sustainable running pace is your goal.

Post Race Syndrome.

Some people experience a letdown shortly after a race. Despite training for several months for your first 5K race, you will not experience this letdown, because you'll be out running an easy 4 to 5 miles the nest day or perhaps 48 hours after the race, and continue to run 4 to 5 days per week thereafter. You also have another race planned for next month, so enjoy the high from this race while recovering. Then ease in some gentle speed running toward the end of the first week and be back to full training after 10 days. Train moderately hard for another three weeks and rest up for the next race.

Additional racing tips:

* Run at your pace. Don't get dragged along to a fast start by a friend or you'll suffer later.

* Run almost even pace. You'll still be working harder in the last mile, but at least the first mile will seem easy. In your first few races start a little slower than you could manage for the entire race and speed up for the last mile to make it a more positive experience.

* Then you can race for personal records; next year you can run personal records on a particular course. Most of us run slower on hilly courses which have many turns. The essentially flat 4 turn race may be a dream, but would lead to faster times. Don't compare its time to a hilly course.

* Race at One mile to 10K, but train at those paces in the weeks before the race.

* Develop a mantra for the moment in a race that you hurt. Provided your pace is appropriate, a mantra will see you through a difficult patch: Sclf-talk can promote excellent running techniques or make you run too fast too early. Include these themes.

o I did long repeats in training at 10 seconds per mile faster, so…This is easy; This is easy;
o I did longer runs in training so…this race is short;
o I'm in shape and I rested up;
o My legs are strong;

o   I want to race;
o   My running is smooth (because I practiced economical running in training).
o   My lungs are huge;
o   My heart is strong…and so is my mind;
o   I'm tall and sexy;
o   I'm short and virile;

I did the first mile at ideal pace, so:
o   I'll keep going strongly;
o   Continue with good running form;
o   Avoid wasted energy;
o   No weaving;
o   No sudden pace changes;
o   In the first mile of the race your mantra maybe "I have more to give" or "I can run faster." However, your response should be along the lines of "but I will save some of my energy for later by running even pace."

Spectators are likely to shout "looking good" to you. Practice economical form to look as good as your body will let you.

During training your mantra may be: "I've been here before but I'll do one more repeat at this pace." "This will help my racing."

When the third 800 of 5 times 800 meters feels easy and you're tempted to speed up the response could be, "I'm at the right pace for today, so I'll save it for tomorrows 8 mile run."

On race day it becomes, "I'll race one more mile at this speed."

Mental training is important for fast racing because it helps you through the tough spots. Run at the correct pace for you on race day, and break the race into sections while controlling the things that you can control. Some days, a racer will run across your path and mess up your rhythm. Let the anger go. Regain your form and cruise along effortlessly while waiting for him to fade.

Race every 4 to 6 weeks at a variety of distances up to 10K. Include local cross-country, road, and track races. After a few months, move onto Chapters 10 and 11; you can also consider increasing your training along the lines of *10K & 5K Running, Training & Racing*. Chapter 14 is adapted from that book.

Chapter Ten

Hill Training

Which will take your running to new highs and to new heights!

If the first nine chapters gave you a Bachelors degree in 5K Fitness Running, this chapter will give you your Masters.

After following the first nine Chapters of training and a few 5K races, there are three main ways to improve your running:

* Get your muscles stronger with hill repeats and weight training so that your muscle fibers are bigger and can sustain high intensity exercise for a longer period. Well done if you've been doing twice a week weight training for the last six months.

* Run for greater distances, i.e. for a longer period of time to improve your endurance and running economy. Kudos if you began to increase your long run three or four months ago. Wear a water bottle holder with a 24 ounce container for runs of over 40 minutes. Include carbs if you're going over 70 minutes.

* Do portions of your mileage at relatively high intensity, including hill repeats and Chapter 11s Interval training.

Long runs teach your cells to adapt: Your mitochondria will synthesize more ATP to fuel your movement. Add 5 minutes to your longest run every other week and you can be doing 80 minute runs after 16 weeks. Exercise physiologist David Costill has reported a 12 percent increase in VO2 max with steady running. Alternate 80 minute runs with 60 minute runs on Sundays and you'll show huge improvements to your oxygen take-up and distribution systems. Your VO2 maximum will improve. To keep running for that long, your stride length will probably decrease and you'll force yourself to land gently. Maintain the same legspeed and your running efficiency will also improve.

To make the greatest gains to your oxygen uptake you'll need to do most of your easy running at 75 percent of maximum heartrate instead of the old 60 percent guideline. It will probably be one to 1.5 minutes per mile slower than 5K pace, so gradually change up the pace of your easy running. You can still do your first mile at 60 percent of max heartrate as your warmup, but then increase legspeed until your heart is at 75 percent of its current maximum.

As the New Zealand coach of several Olympic Medalists, Arthur Lydiard said, "Hill training builds power and endurance." Lydiard emphasized hill repeats after a gradual build-up of steady running: As you are nearly half-way through this book, so will we!

Lydiard had good company. Percy Cerutty, the equally successful Australian coach said that, "resistance training in the form of sand and hills is too important to be ignored." Cerutty had his athletes run up huge sand dunes.

You don't have to hurt during hill repeats.

Hill repeats are not just for Olympic champions. They are not even painful...provided you follow the guidelines of the next few pages. Hill repeats will improve your 5Ks though, while also reducing your risk of injury.

Hill training builds muscle strength, speed and character...provided you choose the right grade for your fitness level. Run small hills gently to start. Run steeper sections later.

You've been running hills in fartlek sessions for several months, and you've done a few 5K races by now. Hills are the ideal resistance training for competent 5K running because they'll make you stronger while also developing your knee lift. However, striders in mud, bounding across sand or long grass will give you most of the benefits. It is prudent to do some sessions up a gentle, asphalt hill though to perfect your psychomotor skills (that is, your running form) at race pace.

In **bounding**, you spring off of your toes, go for a very high knee lift and then land softly on the ball of your foot and with a bent or flexed knee. You only do this exaggerated running motion for 20 to 50 meters or up to 30 seconds at a time, and sand or mud are probably the best surfaces. To work all of your running muscles you can go for height on one repeat, then for distance on the next. You'll start with just a few repeats, but you can build up to 5 minutes worth if you like them.

The ideal effort to run your normal hill repeats is 5K intensity. You only need to get your heartrate up to 95 percent of your maximum during your first 10 sessions. Start with about 5 minutes worth of repeats, and build toward 12 minutes worth. Do repeats of 40 to 60 seconds for one session, then find a different hill for 90 to 120 second repeats for alternate sessions. To encourage yourself to come back for more sessions, it's important to enjoy hill repeats. A gradual build up of hill training at the right intensity will give you the benefits without stressing your mind or your body.

One day though, you'll feel ready to encounter some hurt. When you've done a session of hill reps every other week for 5 or 6 months you can increase intensity for the second half of your sessions to reach 98 percent of your maximum heartrate. If you were running on the flat, your pace would have increased by 10 to 15 seconds per mile, so you're still a long way short of sprinting. However, you have just made your hill session into really serious training, so only do a few repeats at the higher intensity.

The other way to add intensity to hill training is with longer repeats at 5K effort. Three to 5 minute repeats to total 15 minutes of up-hill running is doable for experienced runners. Do the session once a month in rotation with shorter reps at 3K intensity.

Now, lets get back to your first hill session.

You'll need a 15 minute warm up before stretching and a few 100 meter striders, then cruise up the hill at 5K effort. You'll time all repeats, so use definite start and finish points such as a large tree or a specific lamppost. Avoid points within 25 meters of a turn, bend or junction. Your entire repeat should have no cross streets or turns to help you avoid electric vehicles at 50 miles per hour.

Practice good running form but with a slightly exaggerated knee lift, faster leg turnover and more forceful arm action. Do not sprint. You should not be gasping for breath at the end of your hill repeat.

Walk a few feet as you regain composure, and then land gently as you run back down the hill on grass or dirt if possible. Reset your stopwatch (or chronograph) to zero, and stride back up the hill. Immediately after stopping your watch at the top, check your heartrate to make sure you're only at 95 percent of your maximum.

Another option if you have a long hill is to drop a bicycle off close to the top. Drive back down and warmup on the flat. Do your 5 to 10 hill repeats interspersed with walking to reach your bike. Ride down at modest legspeed and the first part of your warmdown has saved your joints from downhill running. You'll need another 15 minutes or two miles of easy running for your cooldown.

Treadmills make the logistics of hill training a bit easier. Run your recovery sections at zero gradient. Do most hill reps at 4 to 6 percent grade to avoid straining your Achilles. Jeff Galloway suggests staying at 3 to 4 percent. You can run hill repeats based on time or distance while changing the grade at a whim. You can run one to 5 minute hills and your "hill" is available in all parts of the country and at any time of year. See page 175.

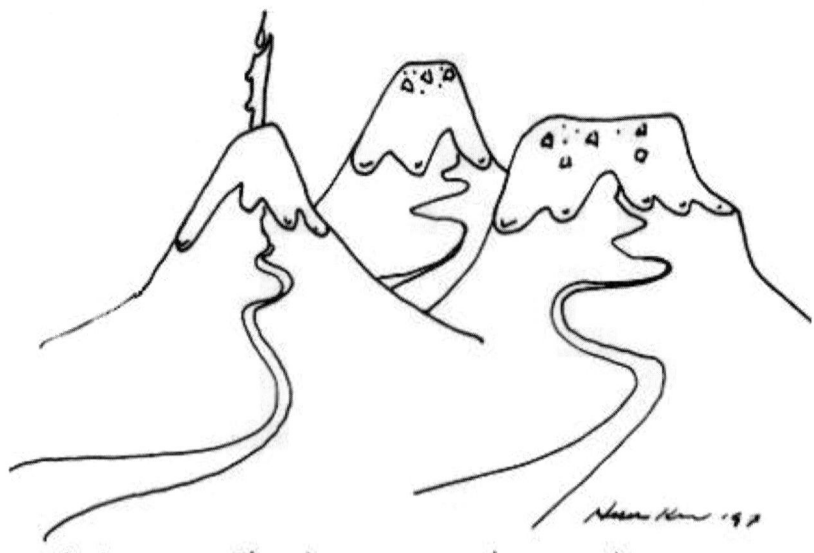

Hills are the icing on the cake.
Hill training makes you stronger.

Don't run hill repeats the week before a significant race. Two weeks before is fine, but do a couple repeats less than usual. This session would be to reinforce your hill running skills and to confirm your strength rather than to make yourself stronger. It takes more than two weeks for the physiological benefits of hill training to show up as improved strength. Running hills too close to your race will leave fatigue in your legs, yet by backing off on the hill session by 20 percent you'll be resting up for a race.

The worst training schedule I saw in the first week of June 2,004 was a 4 week walking program which had its participants do hill training Monday through Thursday. If your goal is to ruin your Achilles, then do the same type of high intensity day after day. If you still want to be running next month, do a variety of training, including hill repeats once a week for some parts of the year, and once every two weeks for most of the year.

If you're opting for a bit of hurt by training at faster than 5K intensity, you should associate with your muscles discomfort by focusing on your body. When you're in a large training group or a race you can use spells of disassociation from your body by focusing on other runners. You still need to use a piece of your mind for the task of running at high intensity, but being with other runners can make your task seem easier. Get into a zone while with others, and practice finding that zone on solo training days.

Visualization also helps during races and training to improve your running form. Imagine yourself running next to a world record breaker with perfect form. Think about how you will feel at each half mile for a 5K race, and practice the art of pace judgment to feel that way.

Good running rhythm will make difficult sessions seem easier...provided you don't make sudden changes to your training. Some days you'll have to kick out negative thoughts about being fatigued: tell yourself you've:
* Run this fast or faster before;
* Run steeper hills before;
* Been waiting three days for this special session;
* Done half of the session; achieved five-eighths of the session; mastered good form for three-quarters of the session.

<u>Downhill striders</u> on a gentle grass or smooth dirt slope are great for improving running form and developing the leg extensor muscles, including the gluteus crew & hamstrings, plus the soleus.

Don't sprint them, but run down a 2 or 3 percent grade with good form and a quick leg turnover. Keep the knees nicely bent at landing and pull the planet back with your toes to propel yourself down the hill at close to mile race pace while making only 5K effort. Run 3 or 4 efforts during fartlek sessions.

<u>Training schedule incorporating hill repeats.</u>
<u>Week One:</u>
Sat – Up to 12 minutes of short hill repeats (the 12 minutes is the actual up-hill running; don't count the downhill recovery)
Sun – 40 minutes easy, but see the next chapter and consider increasing the length of this run by 10 minutes per month.
Mon – Gentle fartlek session.
Wed – Threshold pace for 20 minutes. Do long repeats at 25 to 35 seconds per mile slower than 5K pace, plus 10 minutes warmup and cooldown at easy pace.
Thurs – 40 minutes easy.

<u>Week Two:</u>
Sat – Up to 12 minutes worth of long hill repeats;
Sun – 40 to 80 minutes easy;
Mon – Cruise 16 x 200 meters;
Wed – 20 minute sustained or tempo run at 35 seconds per mile slower than 5K pace.
Thurs – 40 minutes easy;

Of course, you'll also do two sessions of cross training every week. Sometimes you'll cross train straight after your running, such as a bike ride. Sometimes you'll do a separate session 6 hours or more before or after the run.

Want to give yourself a really good laugh? Do your weight training session a few minutes after you finish your warmdown from hill repeats. Take a note of the muscles which feel tired during this weight training session because they are the ones which you stimulated during your hill session. Hint: lift 5 to 10 pounds less than usual and don't rush the repeats. Keep good form. If you normally do 15 reps, do 12s. Do one set instead of two sets the first time you do this back to back strength session.

Stairs and stadium steps.

Add step climbing by taking two stairs at a time for several flights of stairs to give yourself more leg strength. Go down in the elevator and walk up again. Don't allow the knee of your front leg to extend beyond your toes.

Restrict yourself to 25 levels the first time you do stadiums, but walk back down and do 4 to 6 sets. A week later, move up to the 30th or 35th row of seats and higher over ensuing weeks as your legs get used to running or walking stadiums. Do the steps walking two at time with deep lunges; the next trip up the stadium run the steps one at a time. You may need to look down at your feet.

During the rest of your strength training, looking down is probably the worst way to cope with hill running. Looking down ruins your running form, which gives you fewer meters per calorie, and fewer meters per liter of air. Be positive about the hill. Look up to a point about 50 meters ahead to keep yourself perpendicular to the slope, then enjoy the gradient and run at appropriate intensity or heartrate so as not to hurt yourself.

Make hill running fun by thinking about fluid movement as you cruise up the slope, whether at steady effort in 40 minute runs or at 5K intensity when doing hill repeats. Develop flow. Bring your mental and physical resources to efficiently flow up the hill.

* Avoid excessively high knees even though you'll use slightly higher knees during some repeats to develop strength.
* Avoid excessively fast legspeed. You're not sprinting up the hill at 210 steps per minute to prepare for a 400 meter race. Cruise up at 190 steps per minute and at 5K to 2-mile intensity, or 95 to 98 percent of your maximum heartrate.

Do remember to push off rapidly from your toes and whip your leg through and up for the next stride.

Maximum Heartrate test. The early pages of this book gave many options to assess your potential maximum. When you are truly a fit runner, you can consider a maximum heartrate test.

You'll do this session on a Saturday with fresh legs. Do your normal warmup, stretching and striders, then run two fairly harsh 60 to 90 second efforts to reach 95 percent or so of your current maximum heartrate. Take a couple minutes rest and then either:

* Run 60 to 90 seconds up-hill at a pace which gets you to the verge of collapse at the end of the hill repeat. Or,
* Run about 600 meters or 2 minutes on the flat, such as a track or even grass. Again, your pace should take you to the verge of collapse at the end of this near sprint.

Whichever one you use, keep walking. Your heartrate monitor should show one or two beats per minute less than your actual maximum. Your true maximum would be reached at the end of an absolute sprint of 45 to 50 seconds, after which you would collapse, plus you'll probably strain a hamstring or two!

If checking the pulse by hand, count for 10 seconds and multiply by 6. Because it will take you a few seconds to find your pulse and start counting while nearly falling on the ground, plus the 10 seconds to count, your heart will already be partially recovered by the end of your counting. Your true maximum is probably 6 beats per minute higher.

After a mile of easy running to recover from the test, you could enjoy a couple of miles at threshold pace, or simply go back for your usual hill session.

You can also get very close to your maximum heartrate by running your last hill repeat at mile intensity instead of 2-mile intensity (the 98 percent of max heartrate which is the goal of hardened hill repeat trainers). The muscle fatigue from your training session precludes you from achieving max HR.

While many runners do 12 weeks of hill training per year to finish off their winter training, I believe you should also:

o Run hill repeats once every 2 weeks during base training while gaining strength.
o Run hill repeats once every three weeks during a racing season to help maintain strength.
o Which gives a mere 27 sessions of hill repeats per year.

Actually, running can be simpler than that. Just continue with hill repeats twice a month for the rest of your life, and you'll maintain your leg strength.

Chapter Eleven

Interval Training

The final leg to 5K race improvement and to your Ph.D. is to run at 5K and then 15 seconds per mile faster than 5K pace in training.

<u>Interval training</u> splits your speed training into manageable sections of 200 meters to one mile. You manipulate the rest periods to make the sessions anything from discustingly easy to excruciatingly hard.

Provided you did your 200s at 5K pace, you've been doing Intervals for many months.

To give your cardiovascular and muscular systems a bit more stimulation, you'll increase the distance you run to 300, then 400 and to 600 meters at a time. In your early sessions you'll still only run at 5K race pace. You will take such a long rest between speedy sections that the session will feel as easy as the first mile of a 5K race. If you wish to, you can eventually work up to sessions in which your final repeats feel as hard as the last mile of a 5K race!

Why should you train at 5K pace? Interval training will:
* Increase the maximum amount of oxygen which you take in, your so-called maximum oxygen uptake capacity or VO2 max.
* Increase your cardiac stroke-volume;
* Increase the number & size of mitochondria in your muscles;
* Improve the oxidative capacity of your fast-twitch muscle fibers;
* Increase your lactate tolerance;

* Toughen you mentally;
* Make a final improvement to your mechanical running efficiency.

But back to the actual Intervals. As you've already done 16 x 200 meters many times, you can start with 10 x 300 meters. Most tracks have a picture showing the start points for various distances. Your 300 meter start is at the beginning of the back straight. This author suggests that you use lane 6, which is usually the white line (with a number 6 just above it) about 20 meters up the straight. Although you only run one bend for a 300, it's easier on your knees if you avoid lane one. You'll also make a gesture to save the inside lane from overuse.

If there are dozens of walkers and slow runners using the middle lanes, you could use lane two. Leave lane one for people doing long repeats and for the really fast runners.

After your usual warmup, stretching and striders, commence a 300 meter rep at your 5K pace. The rest period after each repeat can be the same amount of time that it takes you to run the repeat. Aim for consistency. Ran a recent 5K in 27 minutes, which is 1620 seconds for 5,000 meters? Your 300 meter repeats need to be in:

300
5,000 x 1620 = 97.2 seconds each

Substitute your 5K time in seconds to find your time allotment for 300 meter reps. Then substitute 300 with 400, 500 and 600 to find your allotment for longer reps. Hint: 600s will be double your 300s time.

Example: 400s for our 27 minute 5K runner will be:

400
5,000 x 1620 = 129.6 seconds for each repeat (or 2 minutes & 9.6 seconds) (His or her 500s will take 162 seconds or 2:42; 600s will take 3:14.4)

600s for a 29 minute 22 second 5K runner will be:

600
5,000 x 1762 = 211.4 seconds for each repeat (3:31.4)

No calculator available in your life? See page 119 for the pace table for 200 to 600 meter reps at 3K pace or 98 percent of your maximum heartrate. Page 140 shows sample paces for Interval training for 800 and 1,200 meter repeats at 5K pace, and for 400 meter repeats at what should be 2-mile race pace. These paces are 95 and 100 percent of your VO2 maximum.

Those 300s for the 27 minute 5K runner give about a minute and a half recovery, during which you can walk or jog, but you'll need to finish those 90 seconds at your starting point for the next 300 repeat. The actual session lasts about half an hour, so including your warmup routine and cooldown you've invested 70 minutes for the 2 miles of quality running.

Make those two miles count by doing them at the correct pace for you. Run too fast and you'll get only a minimal percentage of your training time at 95 percent of your max heartrate. You'll also:

* Waste your muscles if you run too fast;
* Increase injury risk;
* Running too fast is a waste of time and energy.
* Run too fast and it will hurt you mentally and physically while giving you zero benefits toward a 5K race.

Running too slow is also ineffective because your heartrate will not reach 95 percent of your maximum.

In fact, during the early repeats, your heartrate won't reach 95 percent of max until nearly the end of the 300 meters. As you fatigue though, you'll run a higher percentage of each repeat at 95 percent of your heartrate. Do this sessions a few times and:

o Your running form will improve;
o You'll need less oxygen per 300 meters;
o Your heartrate will take longer to reach 95 percent of max.

As *10K & 5K Running, Training & Racing* and the great German coach Waldermar Gerschler said, you will then need to either:

1. Increase the length of reps to 400 meters and on up to 600s.
2. Decrease the rest time between reps to as little as 30 seconds. Cut down by 15 seconds per month to bring the 10 x 300 down to a 20 minute session.
3. Increase the intensity of your rest periods by jogging instead of walking.

4. <u>Increase the workout volume</u> by moving to 12 and eventually to 16 x 300 or 3 miles of repeats.
5. Earn your running Ph.D. by <u>increasing pace for the work bout</u> by 15 seconds per mile or up to 98 percent of your maximum heartrate.

All these changes will make Interval sessions more challenging, or harder on your muscles and mind. Make changes gradually, and in only one aspect per session. As with all running, the key to success is comfort and relaxation. Teach yourself to relax at 5K pace or a bit faster. Your goal is not pain: your goal is to gain better running skills with comfortable sessions, not overly intense sessions.

<u>Try two sessions each of:</u>
10 x 300 meters;
8 x 400 meters (one full lap in lane one, but you can use the 400 meter start in outer lanes);
6 x 500 meters (3 x the straight and 2 bends);
5 x 600 meters (1.5 laps);

Include a 5K race every 3 to 4 weeks and it will take you 3 to 4 months for your first 8 serious Interval sessions, and it will also give your physiological systems a chance to adapt.
    The 27 minute 5K runner can then do the following 4 sessions:
10 x 300 meters in 95 seconds (old speed 97.2);
8 x 400 meters 127 seconds (old speed 129.6);
7 x 500 meters 2:42;
6 x 600 meters 3:14.4;

Note that this author initially recommends an increase in pace for the 300s and 400s, with an increase in the number of repeats for 500s and 600s. The 4 sessions over the next 6 weeks (during which you'll probably race twice at the 5K) follows the same pattern.
10 x 300 meters in 94 seconds;
8 x 400 meters in 126 seconds;
8 x 500 meters in 2:42;
7 x 600 meters in 3:14;
The 94 second 300 meter repeat takes the 27 minute 5K runner (8:42 per mile) down to 8:24 per mile for this speed session.

The 400s are at 8:27 per mile so you're at 18 and 15 seconds per mile faster than 5K pace.

You can then play with the other variables by increasing the number of 300s and 400s by two repeats per month to 16 and 12 respectively, which is three miles of repeats.

Before increasing the number of 500s to 10 and 600s to 8, you can decrease the rest periods quite significantly, though it may take you 6 months to get them down to 90 seconds.

Running at a fast jog during the recovery between reps is the final step to making your Interval sessions still more stimulating. Aim for one minute per mile slower than the pace of your 40 minute runs, i.e. a very fast jog.

Stay in the Training Zone:

The goal of most of these changes is to give you a greater amount of your mileage at 95 to 98 percent of your maximum heartrate. The longer repeats and shorter rests also give you a greater percentage of your Interval training period at or above 95 percent of your max heartrate. See also page 232.

Eventually, you'll include 800 to 1,600 meter repeats at 5K pace, giving you a still higher percentage of your training time at 95 percent of your maximum heartrate. As noted above, you will run a bit more intensely at some time in the future.

According to Russian physiologist, Karibosk, 100 percent of VO2 max is the ideal pace to train for the best results. This is 98 percent of your maximum heartrate, or the pace you can maintain for 10 to 12 minutes of running, which is 3K or 2-mile race pace for the quick people.

Most exercise physiologists, including Jack Daniels, Ph.D. recommend that you run for 3 to 5 minutes at this still modest intensity, i.e. without sprinting. Five minutes will take some of you one mile; for many of you it will be half a mile. For all of you the goal is simple: Get to, and stay at 98 % of your max heartrate.

In your early Interval training days, stay at 95 % of max heartrate and learn to run relaxed and eventually therefore, a bit faster at that heartrate. Get used to longer Intervals at speed and when you've got 15 minutes per session, gradually run still faster to reach 98 percent of max heartrate for the last 2 minutes of each

Interval. 95 to 98 percent of your maximum heartrate is your training zone for effective Interval training.

Bells and whistle <u>heartrate monitors</u> and expensive stop watches allow you to get the splits for all of your repeats. However, it does not matter if a particular repeat is 85.14 or 85.32 because:

* You ran wide to go round a walker on the slower repeat;
* You actually thought about your running style on the fast rep;
* You'll record the session as 8 reps in an average of just over 85 seconds.

You will remember if you run a repeat in 82 seconds or 88 seconds because you'll be hurting and cursing after the fast one, and trying figure out where you went wrong for the slow one. Unless you're completely asleep during Interval training, a basic stop watch and or a basic heartrate monitor to check at the end of each lap and each repeat is all that you need.

You can keep count of repeats more easily if you batch them.
5 x 300 meters gives you a 1,500 meter time;
4 x 400 gives you close to a mile.
Aim to run the second and third batches (or sets) at the same total time or 2 to 3 seconds faster than the first batch. Stay at 5K to 2-mile intensity though because you're not trying to race a mile. Mile pace is not your 5K training zone.

On hot days, you could take an extra minute between batches to stay hydrated, and thus turn your session into sets of repeats. 3 sets of 4 x 400 is one of the classics. Generally though, go straight through your 8 to 16 repeats with consistent recoveries to keep your heartrate up and to experience the appropriate level of fatigue for repeats 5 and 9.

Whenever you can run 15 seconds faster for a 5K race, you'll need to recalculate training speeds for your repeats. Training at 10 to 15 seconds per mile faster than your recent personal record 5K pace is the goal for repeats of under two minutes. Longer repeats should be a mere 5 seconds per mile faster than race pace. When you can run 12 x 400 meters at 15 seconds per mile faster than your current personal best pace for the 5K, while taking 30 seconds rest periods, plus you're doing similar mileage and the other training that you were doing in those 5K PR days, there's a good chance that you're ready to race faster.

Because you run at anaerobic threshold most weeks and have fun with hilly fartlek and hill repeats you can enjoy Interval training for years without getting bored. You don't have to do them at the track. A nice section of grass works well for some sessions. This author has used the semi-rough at the edge of a (too flooded for golf) course for roughly 400s. It's available most winters for 2 to 3 sessions and has no corners. A different golf course in town has a couple of long holes which give almost 400 meters between the tee-off area and the green. While we're less likely to be asked to leave a public course than a private course, this author happens to use holes 11 and 12 of the second golf course for his Intervals.

Treadmills are great also. Run for a quarter mile at 5K pace (again, it's in a straight line), or you can run for time, 60 to 120 seconds is the usual for short reps. Use 3 to 6 minutes for long Intervals. See also pages 120-121 for other treadmill ideas.

Aim for negative splits in your Interval sessions to help you negative split on race day. Run the second half of your repeats one to two seconds faster than the first half, but never sprint your last repeat: it serves no purpose. Negative splits teach you to run economically with fatigued muscles, just like you need to in races.

Take 400 IUs of Vitamin E to decrease aches from hard training sessions, or better yet, increase your intensity gradually.

Training schedule incorporating Intervals.
Week One:
Sat – Up to 12 minutes of short hill repeats;
Sun – 40 to 80 minutes easy;
Mon – Cruise 16 x 200 meters;
Wed – Interval session of longish Intervals, 500 to 600 meters.
    Build toward 3 miles worth of repeats.
Thurs – 40 minutes easy.

Week Two:
Sat – Threshold pace running. Run 15 to 25 minutes at tempo pace;
Sun – 40 to 80 minutes easy;
Mon – Gentle fartlek session.
Wed – Short Intervals, 300s to 400s.
Thurs – 40 minutes easy;

Week Three:
Sat – Up to 12 minutes of long hill repeats;
Sun – 40 to 80 minutes easy;
Mon – 200s at 15 seconds per mile faster than 5K pace. An 8
    minute per mile 5K runner will run 58 seconds for a 200 today:
    Just 2 seconds per 200 meters faster than race pace.
Wed – Long Intervals at 5K pace:
Thurs – 40 minutes easy.

Week Four:
Sat – Threshold pace running such as 2 or 3 times 7 to 10 minutes;
Sun – 40 to 80 minutes easy;
Mon – Gentle fartlek session.
Wed – Short Intervals, 300 to 400s.
Thurs – 40 minutes easy;

This schedule has the Intervals midweek because that is typically when a club meets for its speed session. If the group meets on Tuesdays, your Monday can be a gentle cross-training day, and Wednesday will be your pleasant 40 minute run. Fartlek or striders complete the week on Thursdays.

Run at your speed. Groups tend to over emphasize the 400 meters or quarter mile. Be sure to include other distances. You can run 300s while the group does 400s some weeks. You can run 600s while they run 800s.

Week Five will be a restive week to prepare for a 5K race.
Sat: 4 x 800 meters at 5K pace starts your week. Then:
Sun: 50 minutes running, or do 2 miles less than usual.
Mon: Only 25 minutes, but include 8 x 100 meters at 5K pace.
Wed: Only 30 minutes, but include 4 x 400 meters at the pace you
    ran the last time you did 400s. Example: The 27 minute 5K
    runner who has got used to 10 x 400 in 2:07 should run this
    session at 2:07s. Do not run faster than usual. The 2:06s can
    wait another few weeks.
Thurs: 20 minutes of relaxed running.
You can also do half of your usual cross training up until Tuesday, but do none in the last three days.

Cut-down Intervals.

Much has been written on research that shows fast races from doing cut-down Intervals for 5 consecutive days, either with:
Mon: 5 x 400 meters; Tues: 4 x 400; Wed: 3 x 400;
Thurs: 2 x 400; Fri: 1 x 400; Sat: Race 5K
Or doing 800s and also cutting down from 5 repeats on the Monday to reach a single 800 at race pace on the Friday.

If a person has never done Interval training, tremendous gains in running efficiency occur with the first couple Interval sessions. However, you've been doing 200s for months and also done at least 8 sessions of 300 to 600s before resting up for your current race, so you've made almost all of your biomechanical changes to run efficiently. Thus, this cut-down schedule is not for you.

The cut-down system does have you decrease mileage over the last 5 days, but you rested up significantly for your first 5K races long ago in Chapter Nine. You also rested up for your races every four or five weeks during hill training, and decreased training for races during Interval training, so again, you will not get any additional benefits from cut-down's resting up.

The Intervals in cut-down are too close to your race to give you any physiological improvements. It takes weeks for your muscles to adapt to Interval training, not days.

Even scarier is the possibility that these 5 Interval sessions are the first Interval sessions done by a 5K racer. 15 x 400 meters in the week leading into a 5K race is a huge change to ones training.

Running a single step the day before a 5K race is imprudent. Training the day before a race is ludicrous. The saddest part about the research was that the control groups either did a taper on a bicycle, which is great cross training, but not for this weeks 5K race, and certainly not if it means zero running before *running* a 5K. A second control group just did their usual training without any resting or taper.

Note that Week Five's running on page 114 has you running less than usual at 5K pace on the Saturday before your race. You merely practice the art of 5K pace running. Oddly enough, you'll get just as much of those two miles of 800s at goal heartrate than if you did 3 miles of 400 to 600s.

You also retain a modestly long run to maintain endurance. If you've been used to 80 minute runs, you'll only run for 50 minutes, which classifies as a rest day; if you've been used to 50 minute runs, you'll cruise a mere 30 minutes, also a rest day.

You hardly run at all on the Monday and then take a full rest day for a mini-peak to test your pace judgment on fresh legs on Wednesday. You run a mere one-third of your usual session and it's at your usual pace so your muscles will not be surprised.

This leaves you one restive run before your race, instead of two more trips to the track for those cut-down 400s.

On race day, start your first 400 meters at the right pace and you'll have a superb run with Week Five's resting up. When you really want to peak for a race, decrease the Week Four's training by an additional 20 percent to be even fresher.

Photo Four   Photo Three

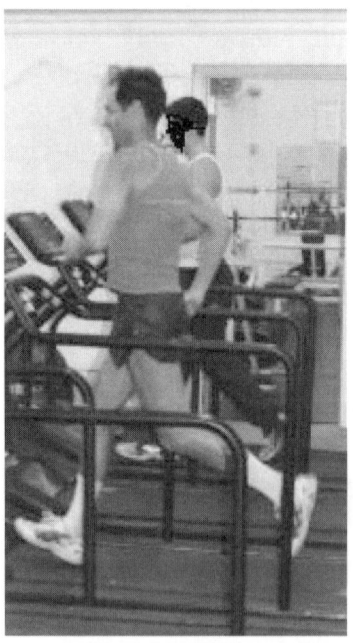 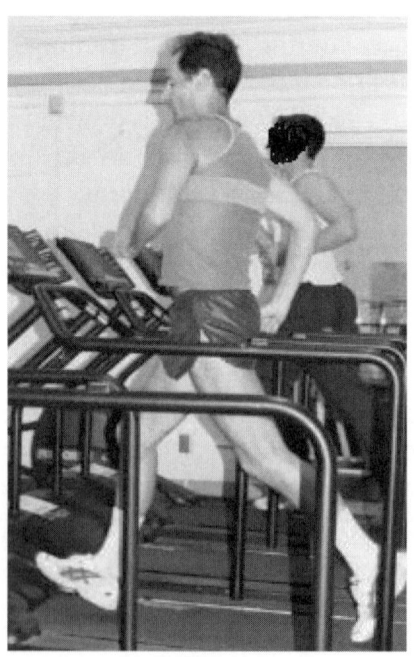

The picture sequence starts on page 117. On this page, photo 3 is just after his left foot pushed-off from the treadmill with minimal left knee flexion. In photo 4, his left heel is coming up nicely as he flexes his knee for a rapid pull-through.

Maintain good running form during Intervals or you'll
miss half of the benefits.

* Keep the chin and eyes level and look a good 50 meters in front to keep your head up. On a treadmill (see below) chances are that you'll look down, which is a drawback.
* Don't let the lower arms come higher than belly button height.
* Feet should remain close to the ground and you need to land with your foot directly beneath the body instead of ahead of your body, which results in a braking action from overstriding.
* Push off nicely from your toes using those well trained calf muscles and maintain a very slight forward lean.

Flow across the ground just like you have in Interval sessions for the past 3 or 9 months; flow just like you will in Interval sessions every 7 to 10 days for the rest of your life.

Photo Two   Photo One

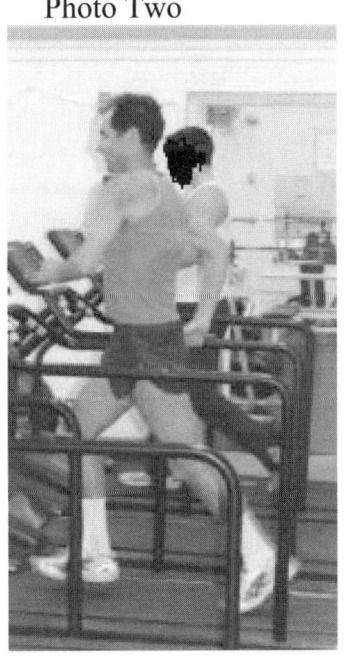
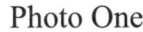
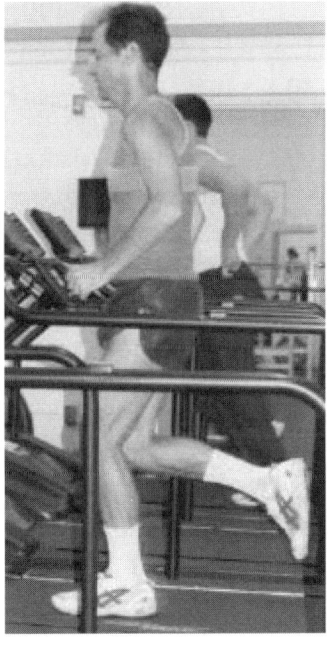

Note the flexion of the support leg in photo 1. Photo 2 is moving toward push-off, with a decent knee lift for 7:30 per mile running, and as boasted on page 118, the right foot is close to the ground.

The runner is a fast (31 minute 10K) shuffler. Note that in pictures 2 through 4, his impact or landing foot remains close to the ground and the right knee is flexed as predicted by Guten (see page 163).

Still longer repeats at 5K pace.

Run 12 x 400 meters and you'll get 12 laps at 5K pace, but less than 4 laps at 5K heartrate intensity. It takes most of the 400 meters to get your heartrate up to 95 percent of your maximum for the first repeat. If you take really short rest Intervals, you'll get your heartrate to 95 percent of max at an earlier and earlier point in successive 400s, but because you rest until your HR is down to 120, it will still take over 200 meters to reach goal HR.

This is why 400s are a relatively easy way to train your muscles for 5K pace running. However, you can get 6 laps at 5K heartrate with only 2 miles of track running. Mile repeats at 5K pace gets your HR to 95 percent of max just before the end of the first lap (just as it does during 12 x 400). During mile repeats though, your HR remains at 95 percent of max for the remaining 3 laps.

Two times one mile will get you more than 75 percent of the session at 5K HR intensity. You'll only do 2 miles at 5K running pace so your legs will be fresh for the next week.

Getting 1.5 miles at 95 percent of max HR is great during resting up phases. Running 800s would take you about 4 miles of repeats to get 1.5 miles at 95 percent of max HR.

Note: Week Five above has you running 800s, but you should gradually ease them out to 3 x 1,000 meters, then 3 x 1,200 and eventually to 2 x one mile before your 10th race at the 5K.

Want an easy session of 4 miles at 5K running pace? Do short repeats of 400 to 600 meters. Want your heartrate at 95 percent of maximum for huge percentage of the session? Take very short rests. Want low track mileage this week? Run really long repeats. Long reps give you a higher blood lactate level, increasing the ability of your muscles to contract in the presence of lactate.

Don't strain to run faster during Interval sessions. As top British coach to Olympic Gold medalists and world record breakers Harry Wilson said, "at the end of a session you:

* Should feel as if you could have run the session faster;
* Should feel as if you could run another repeat at the same pace;
* Should not feel completely whooped."

Interval training paces at 100 percent of VO2 maximum and 98 % of max HR.

Run 3 seconds per 400 meters faster than your 5K speed.

Current	**Reach 98 % of max HR with…**				
5K time	**200s in**	**300s in**	**400s in**	**500s in**	**600s**
15:00	34.5	51.8	69	1:25.7	1:43.5
15:37	36	54	72	1:30	1:48
16:15	37.5	56.2	75	1:33.8	1:52.5
16:53	39	58.5	78	1:37.5	1:57
17:30	40.5	60.8	81	1:41.2	2:01.5
18:07	42	63	84	1:45	2:06
18:45	43.5	65.2	87	1:48.7	2:10.5
19:22	45	67.5	1:30	1:52.5	2:15
20:00	46.5	70.8	1:33	1:57.3	2:19.5
20:37	48	72	1:36	2:00	2:24
21:15	49.5	74.2	1:39	2:03.7	2:28.5
21:53	51	76.5	1:42	2:07.5	2:33
22:30	52.5	78.7	1:45	2:11.2	2:37.5
23:07	54	81	1:48	2:15	2:42
23:45	55.5	83.2	1:51	2:18.7	2:46.5
24:22	57	85.5	1:54	2:22.5	2:51
25:00	58.5	87.7	1:57	2:26.2	2:55.5
25:37	60	1:30	2:00	2:30	3:00
26:15	61.5	1:32.2	2:03	2:33.7	3:04.5
26:53	63	1:34.5	2:06	2:37.5	3:09
27:30	64.5	1:36.7	2:09	2:41.2	3:13.5
28:07	66	1:39	2:12	2:45	3:18
28:45	67.5	1:41.2	2:15	2:48.7	3:22.5
29:22	69	1:43.5	2:18	2:52.5	3:27
30:00	70.5	1:45.7	2:21	2:56.2	3:31.5
30:37	72	1:48	2:24	3:00	3:36

Note: If you prefer your intervals at 5K pace, find your PR for 5K on the left and drop down one line for your repeats. Example: A 22:30 5K runner will run 54 seconds for 200s.

David Holt answers e-mail questions from his web pages at

www.runningbook.com

This one relates to our current subject as a 3 to 4 mile per run person asked, "How do I start Interval training on a treadmill?"

Interval workouts should last for as long as your muscles can handle them in comfort. No hurting because you need to be able to run 4 miles the next day, i.e., to recover easily. Once you've done a few Interval sessions, your exercise capacity will increase, so you will be able to add more fast training.

General running rules suggest you should be doing three hours of aerobic exercise weekly and be heart healthy before doing intervals. Most of those three hours will be spent at 60 to 75 percent of your maximum heartrate (205 minus half of your age if you are fit or 220 minus your age if newer to exercise. Multiply by 60 % and 75 % to get your training range).

If cruising four miles is easy for you, Interval training will allow you to cover more distance and therefore burn more calories, while also improving cardiovascular efficiency. You'll also improve your running efficiency or economy, allowing you to run even faster and therefore farther in each session. Aim for up to 10 to 20 % of your weekly mileage to be interval training.

Fit enough for your first Interval session? After 10 minutes of easy running, increase the treadmill speed to get you slightly above 80 percent of your maximum heartrate (max HR) for one minute. Hint: No gasping for breath; you should still be able to talk in short sentences. Return to easy pace for a minute's recovery.

Then increase the gradient a percent or two to reach 85 % of max HR for one minute and ease back down to 70 % max HR. Then complete your 3 to 4 miles.

Two minutes of Intervals may seem tame, but that's the whole point of exercise and especially Intervals. It should stimulate your muscles in new ways to some degree, yet be fun.

Your next run would be at steady pace. The third run could be two times 90 seconds or 3 times 60 seconds at 85 % of max HR.

Then alternate easy runs with Interval sessions in which you add 60 seconds per week until you've got 8 to 10 Intervals of one to two minutes. Vary the running speed for half of the Interval sessions. For the other half, increase the elevation or gradient so that you change your stride cycle. Keep the hill intervals comfortable...no leaning or stressing out.

Consolidate at 10 minutes per session and at 85 % of max HR for a few weeks to allow your shins and other fragile parts to get used to fast running, then you can graduate to true Interval running by alternating:

A: Shortish repeats at up to 95 % of Max HR. Do the same repeats you've been doing, but after half of a session, increase speed by a 15 to 20 seconds per mile to get your HR up to 90 % of max. Do two repeats, and then finish with a couple at 85 % of max HR.

Start each Interval session with a couple at 85 % max HR, but gradually change the rest of them to faster running alternating with steeper hills at 90 % max HR. Put your legs through a full range of motion with relaxed running form, and after about 10 sessions, you should be running all repeats at 90 % of max HR.

Consolidate again for a few weeks. When you can complete the 90 % of max HR Intervals without muscle aches afterwards, ease the speed up to 95 % of Max HR in the same way as before, i.e., only for a couple of repeats, then transition to faster running for all repeats over several weeks. This should be 5K race pace intensity, but you're only doing it for one to two minutes at a time.

B: Longer repeats at 85 % max HR. (See also Chapters 7 & 8) Match every session of the short Intervals at fairly high intensity with long Interval runs at more modest intensity. Stay at 85 % max HR, but for much longer per repetition. Four times three minutes, three times four minutes, two times 5 minutes with a two to three minute recovery of easier running work well, and they train your aerobic system to work at its maximum capacity. This type of running will push back your anaerobic threshold, the point at which you produce huge amounts of lactic acid.

You should find that the speed for these long Intervals, often called tempo running, is 25 to 35 seconds per mile slower than your shorter Interval speed is at 95 % max HR. You could also think of those short Intervals as being 30 seconds per mile faster than your long Intervals! Each session has its own purpose so:

For every 4 runs, try two easy runs and one session each of long Intervals and short Intervals. Speed training and long runs increase the enzyme activity in your mitochondria, improving the availability of oxygen for faster 5Ks.

Chapter Twelve

16 to 26 WEEK SCHEDULE

FOR YOUR 5K RACE

At 12 to 16 miles per week!

The three mile timed run typical of most military, police, fire and other public safety departments is not a challenge to the recreational runner who has eased through this book. The test can be tough on non-runners because they are:

* In poor overall shape;
* Somewhat muscle bound in the upper body;
* Often overweight;
* Better at strength or anaerobic activities;
* As 85 % of adults in the U.S. can't even run 3 miles, this program will be useful for millions of people.

Poor fitness level.
Don't kid yourself. You know how often you've exercised in the last 9 months or in the many years since kindergarten. Read Chapter One, then get your gluteal (butt) muscles and the rest of your body out there, and start at the level which won't kill you. Build up to three to four miles of easy running, four times a week.

Naturally muscle bound.

The other aspects of a fitness test will be easy. While getting ready for the timed run, ease back on any gym or weight training. Use your arms to practice an economical running style.

Overweight.

Consume fewer calories than you burn but a decent supply of carbohydrates, and see Appendix II.

Fast twitch muscle fibers.

These can be taught to work many times for endurance, instead of a few times for speed. The steady runs will educate them to some degree.

After at least a month of steady running you can move onto the interval work of Chapters 5 to 7, plus Chapter 11...a type of training which has been around for decades, yet still isn't used by most militaries. (Sprinting does not count as Interval training)

The Four day per week training program.

Start with 4 to 6 weeks of running 3 to 4 miles or up to 40 minutes on 4 days a week to get some basic fitness. Run at easy pace. Keep your heartrate between 130 and 160. Then gently introduce fast running twice a week. By:

Running an easy mile. Then run twelve times one hundred yards; use meters if you prefer. Do them at a good pace, but much slower than an all out sprint. Jog or walk for 30 seconds between striders to catch your breath. Run easy to complete your 3 to 4 miles to finish off. Next time, do 16 efforts. Alternate these interval sessions with an easy run, so that you run fast twice a week.

After four sessions of 100s, do two sessions of 200s...eight efforts the first time, 12 the second. Then for two more weeks:

Day one...20 x 100 meters
Day two...easy run
Day three...16 x 200 meters
Day four...easy run

For the final six weeks before the test, keep the two easy runs. The third session, do eight 200s plus ten 100s. Do it as a continuous run with 50 meters of easy running between efforts.

The key session each week will be long efforts. Your preparation should include 800s, 1,200s and 1,600s. These are roughly half-mile, three quarter mile and mile repeats.

Week One: 3 x 800 meters at 10 seconds per mile faster than target pace for your test. This will improve your running form and increase your maximum oxygen assimilation ability; it'll open up your lungs. Take a good rest between efforts. If it matters to you, this is 100 percent of your VO2 maximum pace, or about the speed at which you could race 2 miles. Chapter 11 has more details.

Week Two: 2 x one mile at 20 seconds per mile slower than target pace. Doesn't sound right, does it, but World record breakers train at this pace. It will be slightly faster than your anaerobic threshold pace, which as Ph.D.s say, helps you to run a 5K better, despite running these sessions slower than target pace. Actually, the threshold is closer to 30 seconds per mile slower than test pace, but I want you to keep this session closer to your target pace.

Week Three: 3 x 1,200 at target pace. This is to check your pace judgment. If you get the first lap wrong, make half the adjustment in the next lap, and get it close to perfect on the last lap. Five minutes should be enough rest after each repeat.

Week Four: 4 x 800 as for week one.

Week Five: Repeat week two. It's ten to fourteen days until the test. Don't increase your training this week. Don't overtrain. Practice the art of relaxing at this speed. Reduce the other speed session to 6 x 200 plus 6 x 100.

Week Six: Only two 1,200s at target pace to rest up. And,
Cut a mile off of each easy run.
Day four do 4 x 200 plus 4 x 100

This resting up or peaking for the race avoids over-training...still a common problem of public safety test takers. Rest will give you a 10 percent increase in your potential performance, meaning that you'll begin serious hurting at two and a quarter miles instead of at one and a quarter. You have a greater chance of success if rested.

Note: Those mile repeats were at about 10-kilometer race pace. People training six days a week will usually do this session at 15K pace, or another 15 seconds per mile slower, but they'll do four or five of them. Every other session, they will do the four miles as a continuous run. Sounds like Chapter 7 and 8!

The 1,200s are target pace for pace judgment, confidence and it happens to be 5K pace, which is close enough to VO2 max to get most of its benefits.

The 800s are at VO2 maximum, that is, two mile race pace. Heart, lungs and the rest of the circulatory system work at their maximum capacity to achieve this speed. Nevertheless, you'll still go into oxygen debt.

Summary: If you have 16 weeks before your race.

At least four weeks of steady running to get your heart ready for:
Five weeks of twice weekly short intervals...100s and 200s; then:
Six weeks of long repetitions.

Weeks 1 to 4...run 3 to 4 miles easy on 4 days per week. Then:

	Sun	Tues	Thurs	Sat
Wk 5...	4E	12 x 100	4E	16 x 100
Wk 6...	4E	16 x 100	4E	20 x 100
Wk 7...	4E	8 x 200	4E	12 x 200
Wk 8...	4E	20 x 100	4E	16 x 200
Wk 9A...	4E	20 x 100	4E	16 x 200
Wk 10...	4E	20 x 100	4E	3 x 800 meters
Wk 11...	4E	16 x 200	4E	2 x one mile
Wk 12...	4E	20 x 100	4E	3 x 1,200 meters
Wk 13...	4E	16 x 200	4E	4 x 800 meters
Wk 14...	4E	20 x 100	3E	2 x one mile
Wk 15...	4E	12 x 200	3E	2 x 1,200 meters
Wk 16...	3E	8 x 200	2E	Time trial or 5K

Got Six months?

As above but after week 9A, add five weeks of hills or other resistance training once a week, (weeks 9B to 9F on page 126) while maintaining one session of short repeats. Read Chapter Ten.

Then, do at least five weeks of Intervals. See Chapter Eleven. Do 400s and 300 meter repeats once every two weeks at 10 seconds per mile faster than 5K pace; on alternate weeks, do 600 meter reps at 5 seconds per mile faster than 5K pace.

Depending on how harsh you'd like your training to be, you can run hills or the 100s and 200s for your other speed session during this 5 week phase. Running hills every two weeks works well for most runners because you'll continue to get stronger (weeks G to K below). Finish with the six weeks of long repetitions, (weeks 10 to 16 on page 125) which will actually be weeks 20 to 26 for you. For those of you doing the 26 week option, it would be prudent to run hills instead of 100s in weeks 12 and 14 of page 125 (actually, weeks 22 and 24 for you) to maintain your leg strength.

You can also race a 5K once a month instead of the Saturday session.

Weeks One to 9A as above, then:

	Sun	*Tues*	*Thurs*	*Sat*
Wk 9B...	4E	20 x 100	4E	8 x 60 second hill
Wk 9C...	4E	16 x 200	4E	4 x 2 minute hill
Wk 9D...	4E	20 x 100	4E	10 x 60 second hill
Wk 9E...	4E	16 x 200	4E	5 x 2 minute hill
Wk 9F...	4E	20 x 100	4E	10 x 60 second hill
Wk 9G...	4E	16 x 200	4E	4 x 400 & 3 x 300 meters
Wk 9H...	4E	Hill reps	4E	5 x 600 meters
Wk 9 I...	4E	16 x 200	4E	4 x 400 & 5 x 300 meters
Wk 9J...	4E	Hill reps	4E	6 x 600 meters
Wk 9K...	4E	16 x 200	4E	5 x 400 & 5 x 300 meters

Then you'll do weeks 10 to 16 as on page 125, though they will actually be weeks 20 to 26 for you.

Is a 5K race still too much for you? Start the 5K at a slower pace because then it will not hurt you. You stay in control. Or enter a street mile race. Most cities have them. Do the training from the prior pages while also doing some striders at about mile race pace, then make sure that you run the first quarter of a mile in your race at a sensible pace. This way you'll enjoy the second quarter mile and perhaps the last quarter as you stride to the finish. The real hurting, if you race really fast, occurs in the third quarter of a race.

Chapter Thirteen

SCHEDULE FOR THE MILLIONS

RACE ON 15 MILES A WEEK

This section is for the 5 million people in the U.S. who currently run 250-999 miles per year. You'll see that the times of day at which to train are adapted from Chapter One. This is an alternative way to bring in quality running.

Here, you'll do a four or five-mile run over the weekend, this schedule has it on Saturday, which is the same day that most races occur. This leaves you three to four miles for each midweek run. It doesn't matter which days you run, but as with Chapter One, Monday lunch time, Tuesday evening, and Thursday pre-work allows you to spread the load while experiencing a variety of run locations. You can exercise close to work, on the way home from work and close to home, thus avoiding the "same old, same old" routes which many people do.

You may have already laid the foundations to your running with years of 10 to 20 miles per week. Our simple aim is to do a mile of quality per mid-week run. *You will replace one mile of steady running with a mile of faster running every four months.* You will end the year doing three miles fast each week and 12 miles at your easy pace.

As a 15 mile a week runner, you've achieved many of the health goals from exercise...especially if you also ride a bike once or twice a week and do weight training! While you may increase the health benefits by running for 40 minutes six days a week, it is not the main concern of this Chapter.

The thrust of this section is to get you closer to your racing potential. Early morning, lunch time or pre-dinner runs with a quality mile, demand no more time than the easy four miles you've been used to. If you can get out the door to do a four miler...you can enjoy a mile of quality too.

Goal One: add a Chapter Five session.

On any set Monday, about four months before a 5K race, and after an easy mile warmup, stride eight times 100 meters with easy running of 100 meters rest between each effort. That's it...it's that simple, but do not sprint.

The exact distance does not matter. Run eight times 20 to 30 seconds if you prefer, or lamppost-to-lamppost alternating fast with slow. Note the running form guide in Chapters Five and Six. These striders will improve your running economy and will make you run more efficiently with lower injury risk.

On the second Monday, run four times 200 meters or about 45 to 60 seconds; or run for two to three lampposts. Jog the same distance for your recovery.

The third Monday, do three times 300 meters, or up to 90 seconds.

On the fourth week, run a 300, a 200 and three at 100.

For your second month of speed running, increase to:

12 x 100;

6 x 200;

4 x 300;

Then, a 300, 3 x 200 & 3 x 100.

Month three run sessions of 16 x 100; 8 x 200; 5 x 300;

And 3 x 300, 3 x 200, 3 x 100.

You now have your first mile of speedwork. Take a restive week with 40 percent less running and do that 5K race. Beware of starting out too fast. Your relearned speed will need to be kept in check for the first mile; think about your running style.

For the next 9 months, as you add other speed sessions, retain this Monday session. Rotate the month three sessions; the order is not important.

Goal Two is from Chapter Seven.

One and a half weeks after your first race, it will be time to add a second mile of quality. We'll recruit this from Chapter Seven. You will do it on the Thursday, some 12 days post race. After an easy mile plus some stretching, run a half-mile effort quite fast, or run four minutes. Do whichever is longest. Run 30 seconds per mile slower than the average pace you achieved in your 5K race.

The second week, run 2 x two-and-a-half minutes, or 2 x 400 meters.

The third week, run two times 600 meters.

The fourth, try a 1,200 meter or a three quarter mile effort...but not more than 8 minutes at speed.

These must not be time-trials. Your pace should be easy to achieve and maintain for these modest distances.

Take a one minute rest between efforts.

For the second month for this type of running, you can increase the pace by 10 seconds per mile for the 400s and 600s toward and eventually to reach 5K pace to improve your VO2 maximum and running form. Keep the longer reps at much slower than 5K pace to improve your anaerobic threshold. In month 5 (since starting speed running) your sessions are:

A half mile with three minutes rest, followed by a quarter mile.

3 x 400 meters or 2½ minutes

2 x 600 meters

1,200 meters or go up to 10 minutes.

The sixth and subsequent months progress to sessions of:

4 x 400 at 5K pace;

2 x 800 at 30 seconds per mile slower than 5K pace;

3 x 600 at 5K pace;

One Mile or 12 minutes at 30 seconds per mile slower than 5K pace.

Seven months in, and you already have two miles at fast pace. It will take several more months for your body to adapt to these changes...that is, before they show up as faster race times.

Now is a great time to reduce recoveries to 100 after a 200 effort, and to 60 seconds after a 400. Continue to enjoy the sensations of fast running as we turn 30 percent of your mileage into quality.

Goal Three: Resistance training.

Soft dirt, mud, grassy areas, sand or shingles and snow offer the opportunity to force your leg and arm muscles to work harder. Seek out these surfaces and run fartlek sessions as described in Chapter Five...or do timed efforts of 30 to 120 seconds.

Just as you did with the Monday and Thursday session, limit this Tuesday session to just half a mile, or up to five minutes at good speed. Do this session every other week, adding a minute, or about 200 meters, until you reach one mile: it will take 8 weeks.

On the non-fartlek weeks, do a second type of resistance training: hill repeats...but do them gently.

Start with two minutes worth, and build a minute at a time on the alternate weeks that you will be doing them. After 12 weeks (6 hill sessions) you will reach eight minutes of hill repeats. Use a mixture of short and long efforts at 45 to 90 seconds and use several hills by rotation.

Once you're used to resistance training, try a three week rotation. Every third week, skip the resistance session and do quality on two days only. You can add part of the resistance mile to your other two sessions. Run 5 or 6 times 400, or 3 x 800. Alternatively, try one and a half miles at good pace instead of the mile. The second session can be 12 x 200 meters or four each at 300, 200 and 100. Monday and Thursday would be ideal for the speedwork: Tuesday would be a very easy and restive run for this one week in three.

After a few more months training, you may find you want to do the resistance session AND one and a half miles of speedwork on the other two days. This would give you four miles of hard running in those weeks.

However, take care that the fast running does not total more than 30 percent of your mileage. Adding a fifth run of four miles or increasing the length of the weekend run from 5 toward 8 miles keeps the proportion about right! This longer run would also do wonders for your aerobic endurance!

You can take an entire week off from quality training every 6 to 8 weeks when the mood strikes you. Don't take more than two consecutive weeks off from fast running though, or you risk losing your nice, efficient running form and your muscle memory for fast running will vanish.

Instead of taking a prolonged break from fast running, maintain one speed session per week...alternate resistance, short and long repeats. Keep these sessions easy to manage. You don't need to visit a track. Stop-watch beepers, counting lampposts, striding between stop signs, or counting the number of times your left foot touches the ground all have their uses. Indoors, you can raise the treadmill by two percent for 60-90 seconds for a great session. No downhills either.

There's no need to do more than the three or four miles mid-week to get in this quality running. With only one mile at speed each time, it should not make you feel stuffed either.

If you feel completely pooped after an easy mile and a shower, you probably ran the session too fast. A pleasant, satisfying tired feeling is what you're after.

Keep the weekend five miler really easy...always. While it's no more difficult mentally to do a few changes of pace in those mid-week runs, such as running moderately hard for 3 or 4 lampposts and easy for two, you need the longer weekend run at a sedate pace to look forward to. The longer run builds an aerobic base.

Your 15 miles a week may soon approach 20, as it is natural for you to desire an increase in your weekend run. If you are tempted, don't add more than five minutes, or half a mile at a time. Don't add extra distance on consecutive weekends.

Finally, as homage to race peaking, in the week leading up to a race, cut back to half a mile at speed on Monday and Wednesday (instead of one mile on Monday, Tuesday and Thursday. Cut a mile off of all your runs, and take an extra day off from running.

Chapter Fourteen

Training at
30 miles per week.

Here is a balanced 10 week to 50 week training schedule, adapted from this author's *10K & 5K Running, Training and Racing.* You will need to be a 30 miles per week runner before starting this schedule. Add one mile per week to your total mileage until you reach 30.

Phase One: Base Mileage & Fartlek

You can run one-third to 40 percent of your mileage for your long run, giving you 10 to 12 miles. This leaves you 6 to 7 miles for each of your three other runs.

Your overall intensity level is dependent upon how often you run fast. Two fartlek sessions in which you total 3 miles for the fast sections of speedplay is moderately intensive (the easy running or walking between efforts, though vital, does not count as speedplay). Very experienced runners may only need two weeks in Phase One. If you're new to 30 miles per week, maintain this mileage for at least 8 weeks before climbing to:

Phase Two: Hills & Strength

Hills every week, or every other week, the choice is yours. Increase the number of repeats carefully to protect the Achilles. Run at least 6 hill sessions doing 1.5 miles of up-hill running before cruising onto:

Phase Three: Anaerobic Threshold

Thirty seconds per mile slower than 5K pace, or about 15K pace is relatively easy to maintain...for one mile or so at a time. Run three miles worth of repeats at this level. Run 10 to 20 seconds per mile slower than 10K pace, or at 80 to 90 percent of your maximum heartrate. See the speed table on page 138. Run ten sessions before striding to:

Phase Four: VO2 Maximum Training

Run 400 meters and 300 meters at 5K pace or up to 10 seconds per mile faster...for three miles of repeats. Ten seconds per mile faster than 5K race pace is about 2 mile or 3K race pace, and represents 100 percent of your VO2 max. It is also your maximum running velocity at VO2 maximum.

Run any faster than 2-mile pace and you'll be in severe oxygen debt. It is possible to run faster than your body can supply itself with oxygen because you get a small portion of your energy from anaerobic pathways...the system that does not require oxygen.

French researchers have shown that you can make running economy improvements by blasting out repeats at high speed. That's fine if you want to race at the mile because you'll need anaerobic power. For the 5K you need mostly aerobic power, which you achieve by training at more modest speeds for a longer period than you could sustain mile race pace. Two mile to 5K pace training leaves your legs fresher for your long runs, hills and threshold pace runs. Don't wreck your body with sprinting at mile pace because you'll spend minimal time at the ideal heartrate. Save your body for racing at 5K pace by running no faster than 2-mile pace and at no higher than 98 percent of max HR. 5K pace should have you at 95 % of max HR. The pace table for most levels is on pages 119 and 140, or calculate your exact Interval speed from Chapter 11.

Increase your relaxation at speed and the power in your legs over 6 to 10 weeks with short Intervals, and then move economically to:

Phase Five: Race Peaking

VO2 max training continues, but the key sessions are long repeats at 5K pace, which gives you an even higher percentage of your training time at 95-98 % of your max HR. Cut your speed session to 2.5 miles for two weeks, then do 2 miles for two weeks. Use 800 to 1,600 meter or half mile to mile repeats at 5K pace during this phase. The second time through the schedule you can aim toward 2-mile race pace to hit 98 percent of your max HR at the end of your repeats. As running economy is one key to faster 5Ks, perfect the art of 3K pace running for an extra lap.

Training table abbreviations
E = Easy running...60 to 70 % of max HR
F = Fartlek
H = Hills
HF = Hilly Fartlek
An = Anaerobic threshold pace...15K speed
V = VO2 maximum intervals at 5K to 2 mile pace.
VL = Long repeats at 5K pace
All speed sessions need a warm-up and cooldown giving you 6 to 7 mile sessions.
You can rest up and race a 5K once every 4 to 6 weeks. Note that you never ignore a type of training once you've become proficient at it, e.g. you still run hills while improving your anaerobic threshold (the even number weeks in 11-16)

For the best results, balance all the training elements.

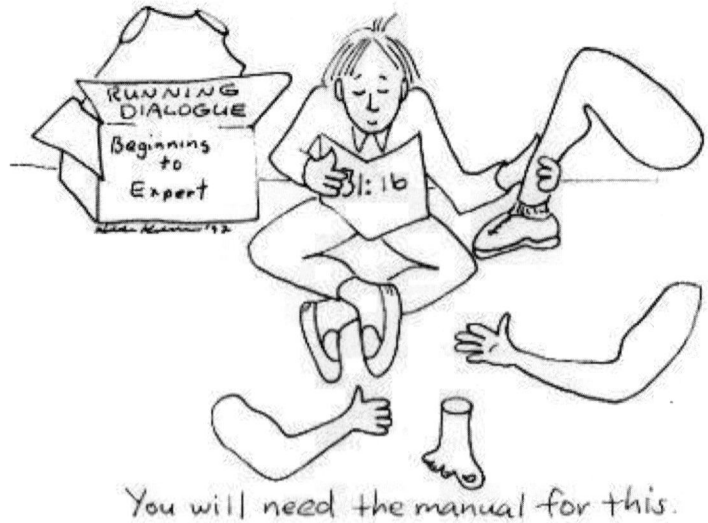

You will need the manual for this.

Use four running days to amass 30 miles per week:

Typically	Sunday	Tues	Thurs	Saturday
Weeks 1 to 2 or 10	10E	3F	7E	3F
Next 6 to 10 weeks	10E	3F	7E	1.5H
Weeks 11, 13, 15	10E	3F	7E	3An
Weeks 12, 14, 16	10E	1.5H	7E	3An
Weeks 17, 19, 21	10E	3HF	7E	3V
Weeks 18, 20, 22	10E	3An	7E	3V
Week 23	8E	2V	5E	Race
Week 24	10E	1H	6E	2VL
Week 25	9E	2.5 An	6E	2VL
Week 26	10E	2HF	5E	2VL
Week 27	8E	2An	5E	2VL
Week 28	7E	1.5V	4E	Race 5K
Week 29	6E	1.5V	4E	Race again

1. For newer runners who have not done hills before, or for runners who are new to 30 miles per week, week 11s training will actually be after 20 or more weeks.
2. Sunday's run is on slightly fatigued muscles from Saturdays modest but well paced training. Save a bit for your long run.
3. You can race every three weeks at the 5K through this program for socialization and training. Cut 2 miles off of the Sunday and Thursday runs, and also decrease your Tuesday session a bit to freshen up your legs a little. See Chapter 11 for the other aspects of peaking for your most significant race.

This schedule can be adapted to 10 weeks by running for only two weeks in each phase; it could take 50 weeks if you stay in each area for 10 weeks.

Don't attempt to speed up those VO2 max repeats in the last few weeks pre-race. Teach yourself to relax at 5K speed. You could include 10 to 20 striders of 100 to 200 meters during half or more of those easy runs on Day Four; you could also alternate 12s with the 10 on Day One. Your options are endless.

Two sessions of cross training each week will also improve your running. 47 pages on the subject are coming your way in Chapters 16 & 17.

Chapter Fifteen

Training Pace Tables

Anaerobic Threshold Pace is about 30 seconds per mile slower than 5K race pace for most people. Running at threshold pace gives huge improvements to your stamina by pushing back your lactic acid producing point, while also improving your running efficiency.

On page 138, find your current 5K time on the left, then read across for your ideal training pace for long intervals and tempo runs of 20 to 25 minutes. 10K pace is roughly threshold pace if your 10K PR is slower than 45 minutes; half-marathon pace is threshold for top runners. Your goal race pace is also your goal times for mile repeats.

The 15K time is the projected PRs based on the 10K time...provided you run sufficient mileage. You should also do threshold training with longer repeats such as 2 miles. Use 85 to 90 percent of your maximum heartrate as an additional guide to the upper limit of your training pace.

One way to move up the table, to improve PRs is to train for that upper line. Currently doing 6.51 mile repeats with a 90 second rest because your 10K PR is 41.15, and because 15K pace is fast enough to improve your anaerobic threshold while leaving your muscles fresh for other running? At some stage, you will increase speed toward 6.39 miles and feel relaxed doing it, and with your heartrate well below 90 percent of maximum. 6.40 is 15K pace for the next level.

When you can run 4 or 5 repeats at 6.39 without a rest week, you may be ready for some PRs. Moving up a line can take months. Try 5 seconds per mile steps rather than jumping up a line.

Don't cheat yourself into thinking you're in PR shape by taking an easy week prior to mile repeats. Do rest up once every 4 to 6 weeks for a 5K to 15K race to check your progress though.

As ever, when increasing mileage, run your repeats at the slower end of your range. Run half-marathon pace if you're in the top two-thirds of the table; run 15K pace if in the lower third. Increase pace by 10 to 15 seconds per mile or closer to 10K pace as you get used to your new mileage.

Do some of your speed running up long, gentle hills based on heartrate goals. Use 85 to 90 % of max heartrate for threshold intensity. Most of your hill training will be short repeats at around 95 percent of maximum heartrate.

Having trouble with the table? A 20 minute and 34 second 5K runner should do her mile repeats at between 7:01 and 7:21 pace. She should also be able to race the 10K in 42:23.

Most coaches probably wish that the ideal training range was smaller and thus more precise. Alas, our bodies are beautifully individual, so you have to aim for relaxed running at roughly the right pace. It will be closer to 7:21 when you are tired from work or other distractions or when getting fit; closer to 7:01 when inspired, rested or ready for PRs.

Running outside is more stimulating & more productive.

Recent research shows that runners will run faster outside for the same heartrate as treadmill running. Indoor exercise can be boring, so unless the weather is really nasty, get outside for most of your running.

Getting ready to race a 5K? Run outside so that you run a bit faster when exercising at 85 and at 95 percent of your maximum heartrate during long repeats at threshold pace and 5K pace respectively.

The main advantage of treadmill running is that it decreases your stride length, thus decreasing your overstriding potential. You can't run through the controls so your steps are shorter, impact is less than on the road, saving your muscles and joints. Your leg speed also increases on the treadmill, and you get fewer stress fractures.

Anaerobic Threshold Pace for Mile Repeats:

PR at 5K	PR at 10K	10K pace	Best 15K	15K pace	Half-marathon pace	finish time
14:57	30:54	4:59	48:19	5:11	5:24	70:45
15:31	32:02	5:10	50:02	5:22	5:37	73:34
16:05	33:10	5:20	51:34	5:32	5:47	75:46
16:39	34:20	5:32	53:27	5:44	5:59	78:23
17:11	35:27	5:43	55:09	5:55	6:10	80:47
17:45	36:37	5:54	56:51	6:06	6:24	83:50
18:20	37:50	6:06	58:44	6:18	6:36	86:28
18:54	39:00	6:17	60:26	6:29	6:47	88:52
19:27	40:09	6:28	62:09	6:40	7:00	91:42
20:00	41:15	6:39	63:51	6:51	7:11	94:06
20:34	42:23	6:49	65:24	7:01	7:21	96:17
21:07	43:29	7:01	67:34	7:15	7:35	99:21
21:41	44:40	7:12	69:17	7:26	7:48	102:11
22:18	45:56	7:24	71:09	7:38	8:00	104:48
23:06	47:35	7:40	73:38	7:54	8:19	108:57
23:56	49:18	7:56	76:07	8:10	8:35	112:27
24:46	50:41	8:10	78:56	8:26	8:51	115:43
25:36	52:44	8:30	81:43	8:46	9:16	121:24
26:33	54:41	8:48	84:30	9:04	9:34	125:20
27:24	56:26	9:05	86:50	9:19	9:54	129:41
29:10	60:06	9:41	93:12	10:00	10:40	139:44
30:25	62:42	10:08	97:33	10:28	11:08	145:51
33:36	69:16	11:09	107:12	11:30	12:15	160:29

Adapted from page 274 of *Running Dialogue*, by David Holt.

The VO2 Maximum Pace Chart on the page 140 is

based on 10K to 2 mile pace, which means running at 90 to 100 percent of VO2 maximum. You should also be at 92 to 98 percent of your maximum heartrate.

If the 400s feel easy, but you have difficulty maintaining pace on the 800s or 1,200s, you may lack background base endurance. Long runs at 65 to 75 percent max HR build base aerobic ability. You may also be forgetting to relax during your 1,200s!

If the 400s feel harsh, incorporate 100s etc., to work on form at speed. Then run some 200s and 300s before trying the 400s again. Relaxed running at 2 mile pace takes practice. Don't let 400s dominate because you can run 600s at 2 mile pace also.

You have to set the limit on the number of reps. You can ignore the 10 percent mileage rule once a month. Rest up to peak with a four-mile training session. Or, ease through more reps at 10 to 12 seconds per mile slower (10K pace). Try 400s at three seconds per repeat slower than usual so as to hit 10K pace, which is 90 percent of VO2 max: half of the reps should still be close to 5K pace. Run the second half of your intervals faster, or alternate a 5K pace with a 10K pace rep. When you've done a particular session three or four times, ease more reps toward 5K pace.

Not exactly on one of the lines on page 140? Divide your 5K time by 3.1 to get your race pace. Run your repeats 3 to 4 seconds per lap slower than 5K pace to represent 10K pace; run 2 to 3 seconds a lap faster than 5K pace to equal your two mile potential, and see Chapter 11 and Appendix III.

See also the Long versus Short Interval discussion on page 141.

The worst speed to train at during Intervals is probably mile race pace. Your heart will spend mere seconds at 95 percent of its maximum as you zoom around the track risking hamstrings and other muscles in pursuit of 30 seconds per mile faster than your 5K pace. Sadly, it takes precious little skill to sprint at 30 seconds per mile faster than 5K pace. It takes skill and self-restraint to run 800 to 1,200 meter repeats at 8 to 12 seconds per mile faster than 5K pace. This more modest pace keeps your legs and heart at the right intensity for great 5K races. It sets you up for PRs at the 5K.

Interval training at 100 to 90 percent of VO2 max.

PR at 2 mile	400s @ 2M pace	800s @5K pace	PR at 5K	1,200s @5K pace	PR @ 10K	mile reps at 10K pace
9:19	69.8	2:23.6	14:57	3:35	30:54	4:59
9:40	72.5	2:29	15:31	3:44	32:02	5:10
10:02	75.2	2:34.4	16:05	3:52	33:10	5:20
10:23	77.9	2:39.8	16:39	4:00	34:20	5:32
10:44	80.5	2:45	17:11	4:08	35:27	5:43
11:06	83.2	2:50.4	17:45	4:16	36:37	5:54
11:28	86	2:56	18:20	4:24	37:50	6:06
11:50	88.7	3:01.4	18:54	4:32	39:00	6:17
12:11	91.4	3:06.8	19:27	4:40	40:09	6:28
12:32	94	3:12	20:00	4:48	41:15	6:39
12:54	96.7	3:17.4	20:34	4:56	42:23	6:49
13:15	99.4	3:22.8	21:07	5:04	43:29	7:01
13:37	102.1	3:28.2	21:41	5:12	44:40	7:12
14:00	105	3:34	22:18	5:20	45:56	7:24
14:31	108.9	3:41.8	23:06	5:33	47:35	7:40
15:03	112.9	3:49.8	23:56	5:45	49:18	7:56
15:35	116.9	3:57.8	24:46	5:57	50:41	8:10
16:07	2:01	4:05.8	25:36	6:09	52:44	8:30
16:40	2:05	4:15	26:33	6:22	54:41	8:48
17:12	2:09	4:23	27:24	6:34	56:26	9:05
18:16	2:17	4:39	29:10	7:00	60:06	9:41
19:01	2:22.6	4:54	30:25	7:21	62:42	10:08
21:30	2:41	5:23	33:36	8:03	69:16	11:09

Adapted from page 273 of *Running Dialogue* by David Holt.

Ready for a change of pace?

Change a quarter mile of easy running each month to anaerobic threshold, hill running, interval training or as striders to practice running form. Make your mileage and track sessions count.

When running 12 x 400 meters at 5K pace you will get 4,800 meters at 5K race pace, but if you take long rests, you'll only get about 480 meters with your heartrate at 5K intensity (95 % of max HR). When running 400s, it can take over 350 meters for your heart to reach its 5K race effort, and give you only 10 percent of your interval session in the training zone.

400s at 2-mile pace gets your HR up a bit quicker, but in the early repeats, you still won't get into the zone until well past the 200 meter point. However, the faster pace is good for your muscles and your running form. You can get a higher percentage of the time at 95 % of max HR by taking short rests between repeats. 60 second rests are the initial goal; 30 second rests will get you a greater percentage of your three miles at goal heartrate.

Increase intervals to 800 meter repeats and you can get the entire second lap at your 5K heartrate goal, and 55 % of your interval time in the training zone.

The table on page 140 shows 1,200s at 5K pace, and they give you over 67 percent of your Interval time at 95 percent of your maximum heartrate. When you've done mile reps at 10K pace with ease a few times, you can consider mile reps at 5K pace. Run mile repeats at 5K pace and they will give you over 75 % of your training time at the 95 % of max HR goal. You'll also be forced to concentrate on a relaxed running stride to maintain 5K race pace.

As mentioned before, you'll also want to run some sessions of long repeats at 2-mile race pace or 3K pace, or 2 to 3 seconds per 400 meters faster than 5K pace.

Many of you will never race farther than 5K. Don't let people pressure you into racing 10Ks or more. You can have a lifetime of fun with the 5K.

However, this author hopes that you do not stop here. Enjoy the next two Chapter's cross-training while racing several times a year at the 5K & 5 miles; if you feel like it, try an occasional foray at the 10K. Enjoy a healthy running lifestyle for decades.

Chapter Sixteen

Cross-Training with Weights

Experienced runners get fewer injuries than new runners do, perhaps because they've found out that soft surfaces, regularly replacing running shoes, rotating running shoes and a steady build-up of training keeps them away from podiatrists and orthopedists.

Despite their experience, the strongest predictor of injury risk for runners is weekly mileage. Whether a new or an old hand to this game, if you replace a few of your miles with cross training, you can reduce your long-term injury risk.

The three pillars of fitness are:

* Cardiovascular training: already covered with your running, but see also Chapter 17.
* Flexibility: see the stretching at page 40. And
* Strength Training, which we will explore for 20 or so pages.

It's easy to rest while bike riding...just enjoy the view as you cruise down a gentle slope, but see Chapter 17.

You rest while running too: Even when you're running a fast 5K you are resting! Not all of your muscle cells contract at the same time! Some of your muscle fibers are resting or recovering ready for their next contraction.

Make your individual muscle cells stronger and you'll use even fewer muscle cells to maintain a given speed. Make your muscles stronger and a greater percentage of your muscle fibers will be resting for each microsecond. Get your muscle fibers strong enough and you may eventually run the 10K at your old 5K pace. You'll also run personal records at the 5K.

Why should you cross-train?

* To make your running muscles stronger, with greater endurance or muscular efficiency...allowing you to run faster with the same amount of effort or farther at a given speed.
* To work your non-running muscles. Weight training will keep you fit for your other activities of life.
* To maintain muscle strength as you age. (Inactive people lose about half a pound of muscle per year, or about 10 percent of their muscle mass per decade, decreasing their metabolic rate and increasing the likelihood of getting overweight and increasing their body fat percentage.)
* To increase blood volume, which gets more nutrients to your muscles, and takes out lactic acid and carbon dioxide faster, while cooling you more efficiently.
* To decrease injury risk while achieving all of the above.
* To take a break from running for a day or two per week:
* To stay fit when injured (yes people, you're still going to get an occasional injury, so spot the signs early and back-off). You can do solid workouts while your Achilles or other ailments heal, or stay fit for life with 50 minutes on five days a week.
* Increase your muscles contractility or power, which increases your resistance to fatigue, or the ability to keep going.

Which type of cross training you choose is dependent upon your goals. Be as specific to running as you can for the best results on your running fitness. Hills and running through mud strengthens your muscles. Bounding in sand and double or single leg jumps during which you land on a soft surface with slightly bent knees give you explosive power to improve your running speed.

Pick up your knees for 6 to 8 striders of 100 to 150 meters twice a week within your easy runs. Don't run faster than mile pace, but practice at a relaxed pace. After 12 weeks or so of bounding and striders, you'll be ready for less specific strength training.

The best type of cross training to build strong muscle cells is weight training. Strength or resistance training will give your muscle strength a boost and improve endurance for hour plus activities such as running by 20 percent, and improve your lactate threshold and VO2 max.

Many people use personal trainers to motivate themselves to work harder during weight training. However, just like with running, you should not be working hard during most of your weight training. If you work too hard, your muscles will ache for days and make you prone to injury.

Your trainer's role should be to teach you how to lift or use a machine correctly. If you can lift a gallon of milk to put on the top shelf of the refrigerator, you have one bicep curl of 8 pounds. Bend down to pick up the gallon of orange juice and you have two reps. Being pushed by a trainer to 12 reps of 15 pounds with dumb-bells and for three sets leads to achy muscles and burn-out. Start with 10 pounds for the number of repeats which you can <u>easily</u> manage the first few times, the last rep should feel pretty easy so that you can repeat the session in two or three days. After half a dozen sessions over 2 to 3 weeks during which you've given yourself zero aches and pains, you'll be ready to increase the number of reps or the weight lifted: eventually you'll aim for the last reps to be moderately hard, and next year you can challenge yourself to greater weights, reps or sets.

During weight training, alternate sessions of:

* Pure strength training using fairly heavy weights. Lift slowly for 8 to 10 repeats. Take about three seconds to lift the weight, and then ease it back down over another three seconds. You should still have a couple of repeats in reserve. Recover while working the antagonist muscle. Example: Pooped out your quadriceps with the leg extension? Walk straight to the Hamstring curl machine and do your 10 repeats there. Then do some chest press or lat. pull downs to rest your legs before doing a set on the leg press machine or some half squats.

* Endurance lifting by using more modest weights. Lift a bit faster but with good form for 12 to 16 repeats. Cruise yet don't rush between machines to keep your heartrate up.

To make sure that you stress all of your muscle fibers, you can hold the weights at nearly maximum resistance for several seconds. For example, the leg extension. After 6 repeats using a flowing action while lifting and lowering the weight every 5 to 7 seconds, on the 7th effort, hold the weight up with your knees at about 30 degrees of flexion for a count of five seconds. Feel your quadriceps muscles tension prior to relaxing the weight down. Do two more of this static type or isometric exercise at 25 and 20 degrees of flexion before finishing with 3 to 4 of the rhythmic efforts. The advantage of an isometric exercise is that the benefit is spread 20 degrees either side of the holding point. You'll be building strength in the very area (10 to 50 degrees of flexion) that your leg is in when you land on every stride. Do a few seconds of isometrics with 15 degrees of flexion too, and over ensuing sessions, aim for half of your efforts to include the lift and hold type. You'll force all of your muscle fibers to work because the keenest fibers, which usually do the initial work, are forced to rest.

Coach Jack Daniels prefers that you only move the weight to 20 degrees of knee flexion, which reduces the strain on your knees.

Circuit training also incorporates weight training. During circuit training you alternate sets of fairly fast weight lifting exercise with bouts of cardiovascular exercise. You could run round the gym for 60 seconds or hope on an exercise bike between machines or weight training "stations". Circuit training does not work in a regular gym section unless it is closed for a group which are all doing circuit training. You get very sweaty when an aerobic element is included and you cannot rush around a gym if the majority are doing "normal" weight training.

Look for a circuit training class or boot training class if you want this type of exercise, or set one up for yourself. After a warmup, alternate 60 seconds of any aerobic exercise from Chapter 17 or running with 60 seconds of weight training such as squats, lunges, sit-ups, press-ups and a few others from this Chapter. There are also gyms such as "Curves" which do mainly circuits.

Slow-motion options
A variation on the lift and hold technique is to completely exhaust your muscle fibers with the so-called "slow-lift or slow-motion style." Do each lift over about 14 seconds: it requires substantial

effort during the work phase as you lift up or pull down over 7 seconds instead of 3 to 4 seconds. It takes work and control during the relaxation phase as you let the weight return to its starting point over 7 seconds. Once you've done several sessions, the last rep is supposed to be a nail biting slog as you work over maybe 30 seconds to do one last repeat. You stay at each exercise for 3 to 4 minutes in order to exhaust that muscle group.

Slow-lift is not for the new weight trainer. This is maximum weight training, can lead to severe muscle aches, and if you follow its proponents suggestions, it takes almost a week to recover from. Their goal is to create such a high level of fatigue that you can only do this session once a week.

It's rather like running 20 miles in one run when your longest run each week used to be 5 miles, and your total mileage is 25 per week. It takes you at least a week to recover from that 20 mile run! If you don't injure yourself, you'll merely suffer all week with achy muscles and you will not be able to run for the remainder of that week.

You will also have defeated Yakovlev's principle. Yakovlev's principle states that your training session must be of sufficient length or intensity to give a modest degree of fatigue, but after a couple of easy days you can easily repeat the session (or actually a similar session). Thus, three days after running mile repeats at 30 seconds slower than 5K pace you should be ready for 6 times 600 meters at 5K pace. If you can't manage the second session due to muscle fatigue from the first session, the first session was probably too harsh for your current fitness level. Running one fewer mile repeat may have been your limit to be able to train effectively for the rest of the week, including the key session at 5K pace. (See Chapters 7 & 11.)

If you completely exhaust a muscle with slow-move, you will not want to repeat the session for an entire week.

Slow lift proponents say you can get a whole body session with 6 exercises. My gym has six exercise machines for the arm and shoulder muscles, so getting the entire body fit with one session of 6 lifts is a wacky idea. My gym also has 6 machines for the leg muscles and three for the trunk. I use all 15 machines, plus a few exercises in the free weights room! One set takes me about 30 minutes. Of course, 30 minutes per week is more than most people exercise for anyway, so slow-lift will get some takers. So will the three minutes per day home gyms sold by infomercials!

Variations include "slow negative-emphasis" in which you'll lift for 4 seconds, then take 10 seconds for the lowering phase which keeps your muscle fibers under tension during the eccentric phase.

"Slow positive-emphasis" is the opposite. You take 10 seconds for the lifting phase, with 4 seconds to lower the weight.

The six exercises recommended by slow lift proponents are:

* Leg extension and leg curl;
* Hip adduction and hip abduction;
* Low back extension and abdominal curl;
* Chest press, shoulder press and compound row;
* Lateral raise and latissimi pull down;
* Biceps curl and triceps extension;

This list, of course, is actually 13 exercises, and you'll need to add the leg press, plus calf raises and abdominal crunches to exercise closer to your whole body. Whether you go for 7 seconds work and 7 seconds relaxing the weight down, or 10 seconds of slow work and 4 seconds relaxing the weight down, it will take you 3 minutes per exercise.

An early 2,003 article said this session should take no more than 25 minutes. At 3 minutes each, the basic 13 exercises would actually take you 39 minutes, plus the time between exercises to move to and set the right weight; it's 48 minutes for the complete 16 exercises, plus set up time.

With slow movement, you'll need to lift 75 to 80 percent of your usual weight the first few times that you do 12 reps.

Slow lift works for three main reasons:

* Your muscle fibers repeatedly fire during your 7 to 10 second lift. They learn to contract on short rests.
* Your reluctant muscle fibers, which let others do the work, are forced to contract once the early fibers fatigue.
* Little assistance from momentum. Starting up movement, or the first inch of lifting a weight is the hardest. Every inch of movement is tough with slow-lift.

* You also get a boost from the eccentric exercise during the slow return to your starting position. See the last few pages of this chapter for more on eccentric lifting.

The lift and hold for five seconds style gives a more modest muscle burn, and you can add one rep per week until it is too much to recover from in two or three days, or it interferes with your run the next day. After a month, add another pair of repeats or a little more weight.

Alternatively, try this drop down variation to fatigue your muscle fibers. This is also called the "breakdown" type of training, but drop-down seems to describe it better.

Lets say that you lift 50 pounds using the biceps curl for 12 repeats and it gets you nicely tired. Like a sensible runner, you could have lifted two more times. Instead, drop the weight down to 40 pounds and do six reps. It will take a couple seconds to adjust, but try six more reps with 30 pounds. If you give muscle fibers minimal recovery before lifting the reduced weights, your fairly fatigued muscles will have to use all of their reserve fibers to achieve the lift. You've done a greater volume of lifting to stimulate stronger muscles. Maintain good form and your injury risk is low.

Use this weight reduction series (or drop down style) for one shoulder and one leg exercise the first session. Two days later, try a different upper and different lower body exercise. For the third session, go back to your normal routine.

Spice up your second week by trying both of those upper body and both of the leg exercises for one session, and do another machine for each area of the body in the second session. Add two machines per week until you're doing the "weight reduction series" for all machines, for one session per week.

Normally take 25 minutes to do 15 different machines? Expect to take 40 minutes for this more stimulating session. Using this system you can get essentially three sets of each lift while only going to each machine once, and without keeping fellow gym members waiting. Two minutes of sitting and twiddling your thumbs between sets is not training; it's an inefficient use of your time.

There is also the **Spartacus Option**.

During biceps curls and other exercises you can hold one limb at the half-way point of your range of motion while working the other arm with a fluid movement for the 60 seconds it takes to do 10 to 12 repeats.

o   For the biceps, that means holding the "resting" arm's elbow at 90 degrees so that the lower arm is parallel to the floor and the upper arm is vertical or at your side.

o   For the hamstrings curl you'll also hold the tension in your "resting" leg with the knee at 90 degrees.

Of course, the "resting" limb or group of muscles is not actually resting. It's getting an isometric workout with many of its sarcomeres firing to maintain the position of the weights. When you do your 12 concentric reps with this limb, you'll feel the fatigue from the isometric part of your session.

After 12 weeks using any style of lifting weights, you may find that you're ready to increase the amount you lift. Don't add much. Five pounds is usually enough, and reduce the number of repeats for your first new session.

Whatever style of lifting ends up dominating, counting up the number of reps you've done is a positive approach to exercise. You expect to do 12 repeats, so get the sense of achievement as you reach your goal. Counting down from 12 to zero is negative. Only four to go; only three to go. It's better to say, "I've achieved 8 lifts; I've achieved 9 lifts." Use the same positive approach for speed running by counting the number of repeats toward achieving your set of eight 600s instead of counting down.

If you don't go to work, you can spend hours with "unilateral training." You use more of your muscle fibers if you exercise one limb at a time. Thus you can double the time of your exercise session for the improved weight training benefits. You will be able to spot which leg is weaker (your non-dominant should be), and re-balance your body if the difference is excessive.

Weight Training for Body Balance and to decrease injuries or recover from injury, to lose weight and to run faster!

You can increase your strength by 38 percent in the first 8 weeks.

Weight training increases your muscle mass, which increases the number of calories you burn per day. One extra pound of muscle will burn 40 to 50 calories every day. That will be worth 5 pounds of weight loss each year simply by owning an extra pound of muscle. You need strong muscles for fast running. Weight training also increases tendon and ligament strength and bone density, which reduces your risk of injury.

Weight training decreases your risk of osteoporosis and most other diseases described in Appendix I. You'll build more lean tissue, i.e. muscle, which means a higher metabolic rate, which leads to more calories burned every day. Your body fat percentage will of course decrease. Oddly enough, your BMI may not go down. Don't worry, your waist measurement, which is a better predictor of health, probably will go down.

Weight training also improves your glucose metabolism, your sense of balance, digestion, mood and sleep pattern.

Weight training does not need to take much time. One set with each lift will build more than 75 percent of the muscle which three sets would! You can also stay at each station and continue with less weight for half the reps as described above.

Should you use weight machines or free weights?   Use both of course and mix in cables and resistance bands.

Exercising at home? Free weights and resistance bands are the obvious choice, or you can invest in one machine with a gazillion exercises...which will hide under your bed!

Belong to a gym? Weight training machines reduce injury risk because they force you to be positioned fairly safely, making you lift with good form. With machines, you can target individual muscles. No weights to fall off the bar either. Machines also limit your sideways movement.

Free weights do offer flexibility, giving you a total body workout. Your supporting muscles have to make minor adjustments to keep you balanced...they'll have to work too.

Example: You do squats primarily to work the leg muscles. Hold dumbbells or a barbell and you'll be working your arms a bit, plus your back and abdominals to maintain your balance. You can work the smallish muscles more readily with free weights. Bicep curls are fine for the ugh biceps, but by turning the hands inward you can give more work to the brachialis muscle.

You do not need three hour long sessions humping huge weights to get stronger. Watch a typical 3-hour weight training guy, and he or she spends most of the time resting between near maximum lifts. Thirty minutes of gentle weight training two times per week will give runners most of the gains available from weight training.

As mentioned earlier in this chapter, there is no need to waste the 2 minutes between each machine or exercise. Do 12 reps of an exercise for the front muscle such as the biceps, take a leisurely 10 seconds to adjust the next machine, and do 12 reps for the posterior muscle or triceps. Some people call this a superset because you're not taking a rest between exercises. However, you're not sprinting at 80 meter race pace so you don't need a rest after a dozen reps. Another type of superset is to use two exercises for the same muscle group, such as following squats with lunges. Then move efficiently to another muscle group such as the abdominal machine before returning your rested arm muscles to say a latissimi pull-down or chest press, or your rested leg muscles to the extension machine.

If the machine you'd like use next is already in use, cruise by to another and then slip in the missed machine later. There is no advantage to doing the machines in a particular order. In fact, they are probably not set up for your particular needs anyway. Many gyms have 6 leg exercising machines together along one wall because gym rats do their legs one day and their upper body the next. You will not be in the weight room 6 days a week though, so you'll do an exercise on the legs side, then a shoulder or arm muscle or group followed by an abs or back exercise and then back to your next (though actually any) leg machine.

You can use dumbbells too. Your gym will have a range of weights, but at home, a couple of 16-ounce water bottles filled to the very top gives slightly over one pound for each hand.

Get a pair of 32-ounce and 48-ounce containers, and you'll get 2 and 3 pound weights.

Feeling strong after a month or so of weight training? Add sand to another pair of wide neck water and juice containers to easily reach 10 pounds and more. Check the actual weight and mark the containers. Still weight training after 12 weeks? Buy a pair of 5, 10 and 15 pound vinyl-coated dumbbells for starters. You might also want a weight bench for the bench press, and ultimately a barbell with a selection of weights. However, press-ups work fine for most people.

Change the number of repeats and weight lifted so that you have several different sessions and greater strength gains.

The Actual Weight Training:

Do your weight training wisely...do many reps, using modest amounts of weight; lift about 60 percent of the maximum which you could lift once but do 12 or more repeats. The American College of Sports Medicine recommends:

* At least eight separate exercises for different muscle groups.
* Do two or more sets of 8 to 12 repeats for each exercise.
* Lift at least twice a week.
* Take a non-weight lifting day after each weight lifting day.

Use free weights to bring your balancing muscles into play, but use good lifting technique.

Breathe in a normal way. Don't hold your breath.

Note: Most people breathe out during the work phase, and in during the recovery phase. Don't think about it; do what's natural.

Do triceps and biceps curls for the arm muscles.

The biceps is at the front of the upper arm. While stood up with good posture, hold a dumbbell with your arm at your side. Keeping the elbow and shoulder still, bring the dumbbell up toward your shoulder, and then ease it back down to your side. The movement is around your elbow joint, not a rhythmic waist or chest and shoulder movement because you're trying to lift too much weight or doing it too fast! Isolate those biceps to develop them. Use a weight you can lift 10 to 12 times, then repeat with the other arm. Doing both arms at the same time is more time efficient, but stay focused. Placing your shoulders against a wall decreases shoulder roll.

You can do the bicep curl with a barbell but it has potential for stressing the back. Using dumbbells while sitting on the incline bench is probably the safest technique. Your back gets support and the sitting angle encourages you to move the weight without rolling your shoulders.

For the triceps, the muscle behind your arm, you'll need to start with your belly in a horizontal position. Lying on a bench works provided your shoulder is just over the edge. Or do bent over kickbacks, in which you support yourself with your non-working arm while leaning over to get your belly horizontal to the earth's surface. Bring the dumbbell to your shoulder, raise the elbow to get the upper arm parallel to the ground, then keeping the shoulder and elbow still, straighten your lower arm through its range of motion taking the dumbbell past your butt. Then swing the dumbbell sedately back round to your shoulder.

Do the same number of reps with each arm, do a set of lunges and then do another set of biceps curls and repeat the triceps too. Build to three sets if you must, but not at the expense of your running time. As with most weight lifting, you can hold the position of maximum strain for a few seconds, or keep the movement really slow: it's up to you.

Triceps extensions also isolate the back of the arms, but there is the potential for hitting your head with the dumbbell. So, use one dumbbell in the sitting or standing position. Hold it with both hands above your head. Hug the back of your ears with your upper arm, and lower the weight behind you. Gradually straighten your arms and repeat. Do your usual 10 to 12 repeats. Use the triceps press-down machine too.

You don't have to visit the gym for Triceps dips. Sit on the edge of your sofa. Put your hands on the sofa by your hips and gradually slide your bottom off while supporting your weight on straight arms. Feet will be on the floor and you'll allow your knees to bend during the exercise but don't use your leg muscles to push yourself back up. Keeping your back straight, bend your elbows to let your butt toward the floor a few inches, and then push up. Keep the movement small if your muscles are not strong; let your elbows go close to 90 degrees as you get stronger. You can also do this arm dip holding onto a sturdy chair.

The deltoids cover your shoulder joint and give you a nicely
padded look if developed properly. Raising the arms up from the

side of your body until they are horizontal, while holding light dumbbells works the medial deltoids.

Raise your arms up to your front and you'll be working the front or anterior part of the deltoids. You achieve better results if prone on an incline bench at 60 degrees. Start with your arms dangling while holding dumbbells and lift them up and out to shoulder height. Don't lock out at the elbow.

Do the vertical arm press (or the shoulder press) in the sitting position with shoulders directly above your hips and a straight back. Start with a barbell at chin height with your elbows flexed and push it above your head to work the middle and anterior deltoid, plus the trapezius. Keep the hands in front of the ears on overhead exercises to reduce the strain on the head of the humerus.

The Overhead Dumbbell Press works the shoulders with a weight in each hand. The starting position is with a relaxed hold on your weights, the upper arms are parallel to the floor and to your side. The elbows are flexed to a right angle, so your lower arms point to the ceiling. As you push the weights up your elbows will almost lock as the weights barely touch above your head (no need to make a manly noise by crashing them together), and maybe your biceps come close to your head. Ease down slowly, and make sure that you have several in reserve at the end because you're likely to lose form and head-butt the weight.

The bench-press or chest press is unlikely to go out of fashion for developing pec or chest muscle power. Figure out what you can easily manage to lift because the weight is going to be just above your noggin. Lie with your back flat against the bench. Push the barbell up and you've got the same motion as a military press-up. Keep one or two reps in reserve, then there's little danger of dropping the weight on yourself. Do the exercise on a sloped bench and you can roll the bar off of you in an emergency instead of it pressing on your wind-pipe.

Using Barbells:
To prevent the barbell trapping you during the bench press, use a dumbbell in each hand. You'll work both sides evenly and you can drop them in emergencies. Better yet, lift 85 percent of your maximum reps: Keep a bit in reserve.

The pull-up or chin-up is for stronger types. After a complete warm up, step up on a bench to get yourself into the up position.

Hold the bar with your palms facing you, and then keep your body straight as you lower yourself down. Don't rock and roll. Simply lift yourself back up to touch the bar and lower your body again.

You can do all of these arm and shoulder exercises with machines. The assisted machine pull-up allows you to set how much of your weight you lift and works the posterior deltoids, teres major and the latissimus dorsi (the huge back muscle). Do the lat. pull-down, pullover, seated row, lateral raise and bent-over rear fly for the rest of the shoulders and upper back.

The Push-Up is the simplest way to train your upper body muscles, giving the pecs, deltoids, triceps and biceps a good workout. As with running, form is important.

* Don't let your stomach and hips sag down;
* Don't strain with your head back or down;
* Do tighten your abdominal muscles; and
* Do keep your body in a straight line as you push your body up with your arms and as you lower yourself.
* Stop when form is difficult to maintain. Don't do one extra press-up, because that's the one which injures you.

Your first press-up. Do some warm up exercises and stretching, lie on your belly with your hands under or slightly outside of your shoulders with fingers pointing forward or inward, which means your elbows are bent. Legs should be straight behind you with your feet a few inches apart to you give a four-point base.

Lift those knees off the floor and tuck your toes up toward your hips. Support yourself on the balls of your feet. Training shoes or barefoot, it's up to you. Squeeze those abdominals in toward your spine as you prepare to lift yourself up in a straight line by tightening your chest muscles and biceps to straighten your arms. Don't lock out the elbows at the top; keep some movement in reserve. Don't allow the shoulders to move in toward the head.

Ease your body back down until your upper arms are parallel to the floor. Get to within an inch or two of the surface with your nose instead of your chin to keep your neck relaxed, and then slowly raise yourself up again. Over several weeks, build up to 3 sets of 10 to 15. Give yourself a harsher press-up by moving still slower going up and down. Breath in whatever fashion suits you.

Shoulders not strong enough for the full press-up? Rest the knees on the surface and do push-ups in a straight line...which means lifting less weight. Or, use the seat of a study chair, or bench for your hands, but support yourself on the balls of your feet as in the full press-up. Table height works too; practice good form for a few weeks, and then proceed to chair height and lower.

Do the chest fly by lying on your back with weights in each hand extended above your chest. Keeping them straight, lower your arms toward the floor, pausing just before your elbows touch ground, and then return to the starting position.

One of the simplest shoulder training exercises for 5K race preparation is to hold a light dumbbell in each hand and swing the arms at high speed as if sprinting up hill. Push your hands behind you and encourage the momentum to carry your arms forward. The emphasis is to push back rather than punch the air to your front. This exercise will help to make up for the lack or shoulder work during elliptical training and bike rides.

While press-ups require you to work your abs to maintain a straight torso, you'll need specific exercises and perhaps some fat loss to look ripped enough for a six-pack.

The mid-section.

Do sit-ups or crunches to help your posture. Abdominal muscles are weaker than back muscles. You need strong abdominal muscles to stabilize your gait, which improves your running form.

Always tighten the abdominal muscles before the movement, and avoid the Ab machines which make sit-ups easier because the exercise is then less effective. Include some twisting trunk curls to work the internal and external oblique muscles. As you lift your shoulders forward, twist to take your left elbow toward your right knee; on the next rep do right elbow to left knee. Cutesy people call these crossover crunches.

True crunches restrict the movement to the first few inches to isolate the rectus abdominis (it runs from your chest to your pubic bone. Lie on a comfortable surface and place your feet flat. With your hands touching your ears, lift your head, shoulders and upper back a few inches off the surface with tightened abs.

A nice sit-up variation is to bring one knee up above your hip, then raise your shoulders toward that knee. Alternate knees of course and keep the movement nice and slow to work on the way up and on the way back down.

Sit ups or crunches work well with your back on a stability ball. You'll be using many other muscles to maintain balance or to stay on the ball. Keep your feet 12 to 18 inches apart to give yourself a three point contact.

Most of the remaining Ab exercises also work either the butt muscles or the hip flexors which help to give a stronger movement around the hip joint: You'll produce more power and a better knee lift by working the iliosoas muscle group. Some also involve the hamstrings and quadriceps.

The seated leg tuck gives the lower abdominals and the hip flexors gentle exercise. Sit back on a bench or recliner chair and close your eyes. Still awake? Raise your feet a couple inches off the floor. Bend your knees, bring them up toward your chest, and push your upper torso forward.

You can do a similar version on the floor. Some people call these ins and outs. Lie on your back and move your legs through these positions.

1. Legs straight, but 3 to 6 inches off the ground;
2. Bend the knees and rotate through the hip to take your knees toward your chest;
3. Then straighten your legs toward the ceiling, sky or the stars depending on your attitude to life;
4. To stimulate your abductors and adductors, slowly do the splits with straight legs, i.e. your feet go toward the ground to each side of your hips.
5. Bring your legs back together, and ease them toward the ground, and then repeat the 5 movements.

Want a nice quadriceps femoris exercise? From position One above do a flutter kick as if you're swimming. The water support is absent, so your Abs have to keep you balanced. You'll probably need to put your hands under your buttocks to do this exercise.

Place an exercise ball against a wall and your back against the ball. Extend your legs out with heels resting on the floor. Contract your abs and tilt your pelvis up to raise your hips and bring your body into a straight line. Hold for few seconds then ease down without arching your back to the starting position.

Alternatively, lean your back into the ball with your butt close to the edge, knees a bit higher than your butt and your feet flat on the floor. With shins and thighs at right angles, tighten your abs and extend your arms over your head while you almost straighten your legs. Pull yourself back over to work the abs.

You can also use your stability ball as a chair, forcing you to make little adjustments and keeping your core muscles fit.

Try these trunk exercises from John Brennand, the United States National Masters Gold Medalist on road, cross-country and the 1998 60-64 age group 5K & 10K meter track Champ.

Start by kneeling on the ground, resting your weight on fore-arms and knees. Raise your left arm and right leg to a horizontal position; hold them up for a count of five, and return to the starting position. Some people call these "diagonal reaches" because you reach forward and back with one right and one left appendage at the same time. Do two sets of 10 for each pair of appendages.

The kneeling back-kick does wonders for the lower back and hip muscles. Kneel on a bench, with your back straight and hands holding the side of the bench. Allow one leg to hang down loosely but straight, then raise that leg as far up behind you as you can. Do 10 to 15 reps with each leg, and your goal can be several sets.

Got a lot of stress in your life. Do the cow. Kneel on hands and knees with the hands under your shoulders and knees beneath your hips. Contract your abs, and then move your left knee toward your chest. Round your back and move your head toward your knee.

Part Two: Move that left leg behind to the horizontal, and then lift your leg with toes pointed away from you. Repeat 10 to 20 times with a 5 count at each end of the movement. That is, a 5 count with your knee at your chest and a 5 count with gluteals and hamstrings lifting your leg higher than your hip. Do 10 to 20 reps with the other leg. Breath in the fashion you find most relaxing.

You can also do a version of the spinal extension. Lie on your belly with arms stretched out beyond your head. Lift the right arm and left leg for 5 seconds, then ease down and do the left arm and right leg. You can also lift all 4 limbs at the same time or do it when lying on a ball.

Knee lifts in the Captain's Chair give the hip flexors nice non-weight bearing exercise. Don't set up a swinging momentum. Make each individual thigh lift count by pausing with legs hanging between lifts. Get your knees in line with your hips or above for each of 15 reps and 2 or more sets.

<u>Pilates</u> is another way to build core strength to assist your running. Check your local health club or pilates studio if you need more details. Eight classes on CD for $23, at reabnyc.com

There will be a chapter on pilates in this authors cross-training book, but it is unlikely to be published until 2,005.

Many <u>yoga</u> moves are strength training in disguise. Sure, the moves stretch your muscles and encourage deep breathing, but hold a low lunge or a warrior position for a couple minutes and you'll feel the quads strutting their stuff. The cobra is very good for your back muscles (erector spinae). Yoga also reduces stress. bodywisdommedia.com sells yoga DVDs. Yogafit.com for CDs.

The Leg Muscles.

Regular weight training reduces risk of lower extremity injuries by 44 percent. Beginners doing weight training for the first time average a 38 percent increase in leg strength. According to top runner John Brennand, "Strengthening exercises are particularly important for masters runners.

"Stride frequency is the same, but stride length decreases with age after the mid-forties. We run slower because we are not as strong. We run more efficiently if the body is stronger." Brennand recommends this upper leg exercise.

Single Leg Drop. Stand on one leg, on a bench or low chair of about knee height. While standing upright, bend your supporting leg until you touch the ground with the toe of your resting leg. Without an assist from the restive leg, push your body back up. Keep the body as upright as possible. Build to 3 sets of 10. After a few weeks, you can hold weights to add resistance.

Half Squats work the same area as the leg-press machine. For both exercises, keep your knees in line with your toes, and don't let the knees go farther forward than the toes: in essence, you sit back with tight abs, a straight back, but the shins stay almost perpendicular to the ground.

With feet shoulder width apart for balance, use hand weights early, a lightly weighted barbell across your upper back when you've become skilled. Dropped dumbbells are less likely to damage you if you lose your balance. Bend at the knees while keeping the back erect. Go down slowly to your knees level of comfort; thighs will typically be parallel to the floor. Your muscles work on the way down and on the way up! Safer half squats can be done standing in front of a bench or chair. Lightly touch the bench at the lowest point of each rep and then push up quite fast.

The trusty Step-up. Using a bench, chair or steps about 12 to 18 inches high, step up with one leg. Straighten this lead leg to pull yourself up. Touch the bench gently with your trail leg, then step down slowly to put your trail leg back on the ground while keeping the lead leg on the bench. Unless specifically working them, don't push off with the calf muscles. Change lead leg after 20 reps. If that's too tame for you, hold a small dumbbell in each hand.

Leg Lunges. Start with your feet together. Take a step forward, drop down into the lunge as if you're in a sword fight. Keep your back straight by contracting your abdominals while lifting your chest. Balance your body weight between your feet; the front foot should be flat on the ground and you'll be on the ball of the rear foot. As with squats, keep your eyes focused on something at head height, which encourages you to keep you back straight.

While pushing back up to the standing position, simultaneously squeeze your buttocks and thigh muscles to pull yourself back up.

Alternate legs or do a dozen with the left followed by a dozen with the right as the lead leg. You can also do the reverse lunge by stepping back to stretch the hip flexors, while working the hamstrings, quadriceps and buttocks.

Lunges test your balance. Take short steps forward and hold on lightly to the back of a chair if necessary. As your balance improves, dispense with the chair, take a longer lunge, then hold light dumbbells to increase the resistance on your muscles.

All types of lunges build your quads to cope with the <u>eccentric</u> or stretching action on muscles from running, and especially from downhill running and overstriding.

Ever wondered why your quads ache 24 to 48 hours after a mainly downhill 5K race? You were landing too heavily on your feet, with long strides which vibrated up your legs and forced your quads to do huge amounts of work (eccentrically at that) to keep you on your feet, and to keep your knees in place.

Practice the art of downhill running to decrease the damage and the work needed to maintain X speed, and to increase your quads resistance to fatigue. And push off properly from the calf muscles too.

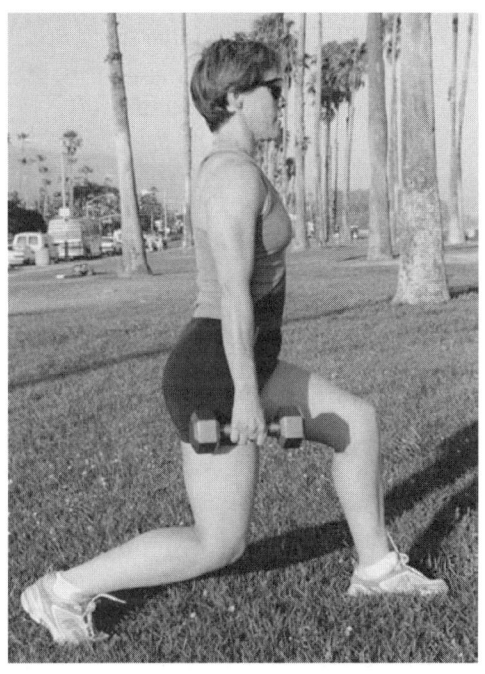

The **Smith Machine Stationary Lunge** requires less balancing skill. Rest the appropriately weighted barbell across your shoulders. Take half a stride back with the left leg and half a stride forward with the right. As you drop down, the thigh of the left leg points toward the floor, the lower leg is parallel to the floor and you'll be on the ball of that foot. The front leg's thigh is parallel to the floor, and the lower leg is perpendicular to the floor, with the foot flat on the floor.

Set the Smith Bar at an appropriate height and you can do partial weight bearing pull-ups and triceps dips.

The **side lunge** will bring in the gracilis muscle and other adductors and the abductors (the hammies and quads work too). Start by holding light dumb-bells at your side. With your right foot facing front, step to the side with your left leg. Point the left toes at

45 degrees, and bend the knee until it's over the left ankle. Keep the torso erect, but feel a nice stretch in your inner thigh as you lower yourself down. Do 10 to 20 reps for each leg.

You can also try plie squats, in which your toes point to your side, feet are twice shoulder width apart and you ease your butt down until your knees are flexed 30 to 70 degrees. Hold briefly and push back up, pausing at 20 or so degrees to do a bicep curl. Vary your bicep curl position to 5 to 25 degrees of knee flexion to emphasis the muscle fibers which are key to your strength in the support phase of running.

Buzzwords come and go. 2,004 uses "Functional Fitness" or training the body for real life, typically combining an element of balance and movement. You do a basic functional movement during free weights such as lunges while holding dumbbells, using your core to stabilize or maintain balance. Standing on one leg you can do bicep curls with light dumbbells, using more muscles, and if it's important to you, burn more calories per minute. Vary the position of your weight bearing leg into a quarter squat or partial lunge and vary the arm movement and your options are endless.

The above exercises work the quadriceps, hamstrings and gluteals: the power muscles for running.

Machines allow you to isolate a particular muscle group. Leg extensions, hamstring curls and the leg press cover your upper leg muscles. Use the abductor and adductor machine to stay balanced. Do the calf muscle machine with knees almost locked to work the gastrocnemious; then do a set with the knees bent at 45 degrees to emphasize the soleus muscle.

You don't need a gym to exercise your hammies. Sit on an office chair with wheels. Sit up straight now! Adjust the seat height to get your feet flat on the floor...then drop the seat another inch. Lift your lower legs and place your heals 6 to 12 inches in front of you. Pull yourself forward, then "walk" your chair around the room while staying seated. Feel those hamstrings work.

The stiff-legged deadlift is good for the hamstrings and their surrounding muscles. Feet a few inches apart, hold a pair of light dumbbells with tight abs, lean forward at the hips and with a straight back and straight legs lower the weights toward the floor. Feel a nice hammie stretch, then ease back up to stand and repeat for 10 to 15 reps.

According to Dr. Gary Guten in his book, *Running Injuries,* when we are in ground contact during running, our knee flexion is about 25 to 40 degrees, and our quadriceps and hamstrings both contract to keep the knee joint stable.

You don't have to straighten your leg during the leg press and other exercises above, and you don't have to take your ankles all the way to your butt to work your hamstrings. You can focus much of your weight training on the range of motion (ROM) most crucial to your running. After five full ROM repeats with each exercise, move the weight to a relaxed knee bend of 15 degrees, then move the weights slowly to a knee flexion of 50 degrees to give yourself a nice fluff factor at each end of the range. Do 8 to 10 slow repeats over this short ROM and then finish with a few full ROM repeats.

Do the leg extension at 5 to 30 degrees of knee flexion to strengthen the vastus medialis, and decrease your risk of chondromalacia.

The gluteus maximus is busy during 40 percent of the stance or support phase and the abductors also work during 50 percent of the support phase, so remember to work those muscles too. Strong, knee stabilizing abductors reduce your risk of chondromalacia or Runner's knee, which is a pain under the patella or knee cap.

Here's John Brennand's favorite lower leg exercise.
Stand on the second step with the right foot for balance, and your weight on the left forefoot at the first step. Bounce rapidly ten times on the left foot. Do three sets of ten for each foot.

Or do...**Heel Raises**.
Stand on the balls of your feet on a two inch block or a stair. Raise your heels up by contracting your calves, then roll up onto your toes. After a pause, drop slowly back down so that the heel dips below the step. Keep a steady and rhythmic movement. Do single leg raises for still stronger calves. Do calf stretches too! Note: Too much of this exercise can strain the plantar fascia or the Achilles tendon. After a few months you can hold light and then increasingly heavy dumbbells to make your calves stronger.

The above two exercises work the gastrocnemius and soleus, which extends the foot and give power at stride-off. You'll also stretch your Achilles tendons during the section of the exercise which is below the step.

When the heel is at its lowest point, the calf muscles should be fully stretched. If you make a conscious effort to push down still further you'll have an eccentric muscle exercise, which Swedish researchers have shown to be an effective way to clear Achilles Tendonitis. Eccentric contractions occur when the muscle lengthens during a work phase. The eccentric contraction produces more tension than a concentric contraction.

Of course, most weight training focuses on concentric exercise, which involves a shortening of the muscles to create movement. Push up very slowly with the calf to make them strong with the concentric exercise. However, push down to lengthen the calf and Achilles to allow them the chance to withstand the forces when you run. But avoid overstriding to keep the forces to a minimum.

The calf and hamstrings do much of their work when they are already at nearly full length. The impact when we land forces the calf and Achilles to withstand huge forces while they lengthen a bit more during the support phase of each stride, prior to shortening of the muscles to achieve push-off. According to Guten, the calf muscles work during 60 percent of the stance phase. Then of course, they have to possess the endurance to push-off during the propulsion phase to give you forward movement.

You can do eccentric exercise when you do most of your stretching. The wall stretch is great for the calf and Achilles, but push the heel slowly toward the ground and you'll stretch the muscles a bit a more.

The benefits from eccentric training may come from:
*   The increased length of the muscle-tendon unit, or
*   Increased strength in the muscle and tendon.

To get the full benefit from eccentric exercise, move back to a neutral position very slowly after your concentric exercise. After you've lifted your weight fully up onto your toes in the calf raise, slowly lower yourself back to dorsiflexion. Your calf muscle fibers will be forced to work as they lengthen to their full length. You will also be working the Tibialis Anterior which is at the front of the shin. The tibialis lifts the foot into dorsiflexion and complements the work of the calf muscles.

The simple way to do eccentric exercise is with relatively slow lift such as lifting over 4 seconds and then moving, or allowing the weight to move back, over 10 seconds for some of your repeats.

You might want to use elastic bands like the thera-band for early eccentric muscle contractions. You'll be using your arms to set up the resistance, which lessens the risk of over stretching muscles. Point your toes just like you would at the high point of the calf raise, and then ease your foot slowly into dorsiflexion while maintaining resistance with the band. Bands are also a great way to strengthen your calves before doing the page 163 exercises.

The calf press machine in the gym does essentially the same movement as calf raises. Some machines have you sitting, so it's easier to choose light weights for eccentric practice; others have you standing, so at a minimum, you'll be lifting your own weight.

Eccentric exercise proponents suggest that you lift your weight up onto your toes using both feet and then transfer all weight to one leg for the descent or eccentric phase. Do the same number of repeats for each leg, but take care or you'll be out of running for three months with a major calf strain. Add your reps slowly over several weeks.

Tim Noakes in *Lore of Running* mentions that due to the rebound energy from their huge Achilles tendons, kangaroos use the same amount of oxygen as they speed up toward their most efficient speed. You have a most efficient running speed too. Your Achilles won't rebound forever, so let all of your connective tissues heal with sufficient rest each week and each year, and run with the right stride length for you to be efficient.

Hamstrings get stronger with eccentric exercise too. When you've shortened the hammies with your curl, slowly ease your lower leg almost back to the straight position and force your hammies sarcomeres to fire a few more times as they lengthen.

Alphabet or numbers and Shin Lift.
While sitting in a chair, raise your feet and write the alphabet or zero to nine several times with your toes.

In a similar position, or sitting on a table, use a weight around your foot. Move the foot up and down at the ankle. This is often called the paint-pot exercise. Or place a dumb-bell on your toes and lift it up using your shin muscles.

Feel like developing calf endurance with your weight training? <u>Try skipping rope.</u> Although you'll work the upper leg muscles and arms, the calf muscles do most of the work. Ten minutes will burn 100 calories, or 5 pounds of fat per year if you do it every other day. Oddly enough, it's mainly the calf muscles which propel you forward in running! Wear sturdy shoes on a forgiving surface. Build up slowly over several weeks and stop if you feel leg pains.

"It takes months of regular weights and resistance training before you see results," says Brennand, "Do make it a regular part of your training."

Don't overtrain with weight lifting. Don't jump into three sets of lifting 80 pounds when your maximum single lift is 90 pounds. Lift 60 to 70 percent of your max lift so as not to insult your body with unrealistic amounts of weight training. Most runners should be aiming for 15 repeats of each exercise because you need endurance and strength. Leg muscles respond well to 20 reps per set. Do a few minutes of gentle aerobic exercise and stretching after weight training to reduce stiffness.

Five minutes on the elliptical trainer and 2 or 3 on a rowing machine is a nice way to warm up and to cooldown for weight training. They also mark the beginnings of aerobic cross training.

Your first 10 to 12 weeks at strength and cross training will allow you to rest up three times to race. That is, just as you did in earlier chapters you'll do full training for 3 to 4 weeks, then train gently to rest up so that your body can make physiological adaptations, while you also rest for a low-key race.

A 5K, 5 miles and 5K would be excellent practice for all runners. Don't rest up very much. Your major peak should be after running a series of Interval sessions at 5K to 3K race pace, to stimulate your VO2 maximum. The races during your first cross training experience are for training and for personal delight. Then, take your leg muscle and upper body strength into another 20-week, 5K training program for several more races. Also, make a lifetime commitment to cross training.

Chapter Seventeen

Aerobic or Cardiovascular

Cross Training.

Add a couple of bicycle rides or elliptical sessions to Chapter Sixteen's strength training...and oxen will be jealous of your power. Develop the strength to help you maintain running form and running speed despite your race fatigue.

As stated early in Chapter Sixteen, cross training decreases injury risk while maintaining or increasing endurance. Whichever types of aerobic cross training exercise you do, build up slowly. After a few weeks, incorporate a series of one to five minute efforts at modest intensity to stimulate your cardiovascular system. If you find that you really like cross-training, aim for 3 to 5 minute intervals at 5K intensity. Or:

* Do 15 minutes cross training as a warm-up before running;
* On hot or cold days do 40 minutes as a substitute for running;
* Do 15 minutes as your cooldown with a drink by your side.

Be specific. It takes quality running to run well. The "specificity rule of training" states that:

To run a good 5K, you must run significant mileage at two minutes per mile slower than 5K pace, and 20 to 30 percent of your mileage close to or a bit faster than 5K pace. Cross training must mimic running as much as possible to be effective.

Your aerobic capacity will increase if you add any cross training, while maintaining your running workouts. However, if your cross training is specific enough, you can also get the same training benefit when using it as a substitute for running.

Cross training exercise goals include:

* Weight bearing: Avoid sitting if possible. Rowing machines are poor. If you stand for uphill biking...fine. Elliptical trainers are even better.

* Beat the weather: Biking and pool work are excellent on hot days. Set up fans indoors and regulate the temperature to use most types of machine. Running on a treadmill is not cross training but it keeps you off the ice or out of the sun. Set up your bicycle on bike rollers and you'll also have cross training away from the ice.

* Variety: See some different scenery and cover greater distance while biking, or have company while using exercise machines at the gym.

* Recovery from runs: Yesterdays session should have been light enough that you can cruise for 6 to 10 miles of running for pleasure today, but you can still substitute 50 to 60 minutes of cross training instead. Remember to mimic running, ensure that it's relaxing, yet get your heartrate up. You should plan on complete rest days from exercise too.

* Reduce the impact on your joints. Land softly and avoid overstriding to reduce the affects of ground impact on every stride. However, run in the pool too.

* Increase your training: Give your muscles extra training while still running your 20 or 30 miles per week.

* Available when injured: Some of your cross-training exercise options should be available if you're lame. Being injured is usually a lame excuse for not exercising.

Because running is endurance focused, after weight training, the 2nd through 4th choice for cross training goes to continuous activities which use most of your muscles. All three options give huge rewards for:

* Recovery from runs or as a substitute for a run.

* Add-ons to the end of a run, or the warm-up before running.

* Non or low-impact quality training.
* And of course, for additional training.

Choose the activities which you like because you're more likely to do them. Fitness training requires consistent training. You need three or four main quality sessions of running or cross training, plus several other sessions to make you fit enough to train long or hard on those three main training days.
The three best aerobic exercises for runners:

Choice One: Deep Water Running.

Doesn't sound like cross-training, but because you've eliminated the ground impact, water running is clearly the best alternative to land running. For most of us, it means running in a pool. Keep it interesting by having a companion, listening to music, or by doing gentle intervals at threshold or at 5K intensity (Chapters 7, 8 & 11). Pool running is substantially more running muscle specific than swimming, and it's easier to get your exercise high.

Pool running works most of your muscles. Unlike elliptical training and biking, it gives a significant workout for the arms: You work your arms exactly the same way as you do for land running! Your arms also have to work against the water's resistance, so pool running gives a great cardiorespiratory workout.

Because you're working your arms and perfectly mimicking land running, every minute of pool running is equivalent to a minute of land running…if your heartrate is in the training range.

You can pool run while recuperating from most running injuries such as Tendonitis, stress fractures, ankle and knee problems. Fail to address the cause, and injuries may return a few weeks after you switch back to land running. You may:

* Need different shoes;
* Need to run on softer surfaces;
* Need to correct your running form;
* Need to slow down to avoid overtraining;
* Need cross-training for 20 to 40 percent of your training;
* Need to give your body time to catch up with your training.

Acute muscle injuries will usually need total rest of that body part for a few days, but many people can then commence gentle pool running. It's easy to strain your muscles during pool running, so practice restraint with recently strained muscles.

Because of the hydrostatic pressure which forces blood back into your heart, your heart pushes out more blood per stroke when you're in water. Your heartrate is therefore lower when exercising in the wet stuff. To get the equivalent training effect as land running, your intensity needs to feel a bit harder. Your heartrate will still be lower. You still don't need to run at mile pace intensity. Gentle intervals mean doing 2-mile effort in water to get 5K training intensity; run 10K effort to get 15K intensity.

Pick intervals of one to 10 minutes and do them at harsher than land running effort. Your heartrate will still be quite low. Run at speed for the same total length of time which you would normally do. Drink fluids every 10 to 15 minutes if the session (including your weights and other cross training) lasts over an hour.

You can work on your flexibility with pool running. Pool running does tend to over emphasize the hip flexors and extensors, while resting the weight bearing calves and quadriceps muscles. This also means you are not building up the calves and quads! Be sure to match every 40-minute pool session with a few minutes of weight training for the calves and quadriceps muscles.

Maintain good running form by leaning forward only slightly or remaining upright with your head up. Swing those arms just as much as you would during land running. Your hands should be lightly clenched and come up no higher than nipple height, which means that they stay under the water. It is probably even better if you don't see your hands come up in front of you. Keep them closer to waist height for faster cadence. Push them back to slightly behind your butt and keep the motion forward and backward.

Do your pool running in deep water so that your feet don't touch the bottom. A flotation vest helps to take the strain off your shoulders and allows you to work on running form. If you also do exercises in the shallow end such as jumping exercises for your calf muscles, use aquatic shoes or old, sturdy walking sandals. You can work the calf muscles at their most important skill...pushing you forward on each stride. Do a few minutes of easy pool running to finish off.

Need a break after half of your intervals? Lie on your back and kick with your legs as if swimming backstroke. Then give the hamstrings a bonus workout by pulling yourself back up the pool on your back while flipping your ankles rapidly to your buttocks.

Water is a great non-impact training opportunity.

Pool running saves your muscles, tendons and joints for a longer running life. You can take your hip flexors and extensors through a huge range of motion, but you'll get no damage from an over-striding impact. Use water running wisely. Don't jump into a session the day before your main speed training session. You can easily fatigue your hip flexors during pool running, so save the pool for the day AFTER speed training.

Think about your running motion. You'll soon develop bad running form if you do high training volume in water. Use a running vest if it feels right for you, though some people think the vest restricts their movement. Vestless running generally forces you to exercise harder. If you're after a low intensity exercise session, wearing a vest is a wise choice. Training hard in the pool? Give the vest a miss after you've warmed up.

Don't restrict pool running to rest days. You can run one of your hard sessions at threshold pace or VO2 maximum effort (5K pace) in the pool each week: The next day, do your easy and pleasure seeking running on land.

Water running is an opportunity to add a half session of training or to take an easy day. Feeling really tired this week? Instead of your fairly typical 3 times one mile at 10K pace or 12 times 400 meters at 5K pace, head to the pool. Do 2 x 5 minutes quite hard, or 6 x one minute slightly harder. For the serious 5K runner, this would be half of the normal track session. Add the fact that it's non-impact, and you should feel refreshed the next time you run.

The pool session could also be done as an extra session the day after speedwork. Add a short, modest quality pool session to your 2 weekly land speed sessions to give yourself two and a half speed sessions a week. Do this only on alternate weeks, and there's minimal over training potential.

When doing Intervals you also get 75 % of the running benefits from the first half of a pool running session! Pool running is the perfect way to finish your long run on hot days. Do seven miles outside, and finish with 21 to 30 minutes in the pool, or however long it would have taken for those last three miles.

Live close to a sandy beach or wash? A pleasant

variation to reduce ground impact is to run though 6 to 12 inches of water at a variety of paces, with or without an old pair of running shoes. Benefits include:

* You have to lift your knees to avoid falling so you'll get a bounding type exercise for strength.
* The water cushions your landing.
* The sand or shale cushions your landing still more.
* The ground moves away from you at push-off.
* The splashed water is cooling, so: You could alternate a 3 minute fast effort on the firm, yet forgiving sandbar, with 3 minutes easy pace running through shallow water, followed by a minute of fast running through shallow water, then repeat.
* Hopefully, there will be a few deep spots which you can fall into. You also have to work to lift those wet shoes.

Swimming.

You're in the pool, so I owe it to you to discuss swimming as cross-training. If water running is available, don't swim. If you really enjoy swimming though, go ahead.

Running uses mostly leg muscles for power and propulsion. Surprised you with that one, didn't I? Swimming uses about 80 percent upper body muscles to move you through the water.

* Used as a rest, swimming can keep you away from training.
* Used to build your shoulder and arm muscles, swimming can be used as training!

Though they are not mutually exclusive, you probably need to decide whether rest or training is your goal. Apart from diving starts, your fastest five meters of swimming is after you push off from the wall...for every length of the pool. Want to rest your legs for running? Push off gently at each turn and pick up speed using your arms and shoulders.

Want to work your gluteals, hamstrings, quadriceps and calf muscles? Push off strongly and rapidly and you've got a leg press against the waters resistance as you reverse momentum and reach maximum speed in mere hundredths of a second. Extend the push off through your toes like you would at full stride for the calf muscles. You can also give more emphasis to your legs by holding a float with your hands for extensive sessions of kicking. Why do that when you can run in the pool?

Going to swim? Alternate freestyle or frontcrawl with backstroke to balance your session. Breaststroke puts too much strain upon the knees and butterfly is too technical, plus it requires and stimulates excessive shoulder power.

Stimulate the cardiorespiratory system by breathing every 3 to 5 strokes instead of every 2 strokes which fast swimming needs.

Swim at easy effort. Just like with running, don't get severely out of breath in the early sessions. Be gentle with yourself until you develop a feel for the water, then try:

Interval Training with 50 to 100 meters of fast swimming, alternating with slow swimming, or with 15 to 30 seconds rest.

Or do 6 lengths at a time. Two of frontcrawl, one of backcrawl and repeat. Breathe every 4 strokes during the first couple of sets, and every 6 strokes toward the end of the session. After the 30 second rest from the second set, try a 12-stroke cycle for the first pool length of each set. This swim session is best done after weight training and elliptical training.

As with pool running, your heartrate will be lower during swimming compared to land running.

Unless you're planning a triathlon, speed is not your main goal: aquadynamics and swimming trunks are out; baggy shorts will do. Do learn how to swim efficiently though to decrease shoulder injury risk. Lead with the top of your head while looking down at the bottom of the pool. Lean on your chest so that your lower body floats high in the water. Don't splash. Extend your arm well forward, and slip it into the water without making waves.

You can use fins to work your legs a bit more, and use a kickboard for one minute in five to save your arms.

Tons of swimming workouts at US Masters Swimming
usms.org/training/workouts.htm

Swimming outside? Turn your head toward land for breaths and to monitor the shore. Stay parallel to the shore. Look up for the marker buoys if your beach has them. Stay close to the lifeguard.

Choice Two: Elliptical Trainer.

Elliptical workouts are the second best aerobic cross training option for runners because you stand for all of your training. Provided you don't place excessive weight on your hands, and that exercise at the same intensity, elliptical training will give you the same heartrate and oxygen consumption as treadmill running.

The movement is a gentle ellipse, giving a smooth, rolling action without actual impact. It's great for avoiding injuries, or to maintain fitness while your joints and muscles heal. You can also do most of these suggested elliptical sessions on a stair-climber, but watch out for knee trouble on the stairs. Elliptical training is a cross between cycling, running and stair-climbing, but:

*   No traffic or road rage worries and almost zero impact;
*   While standing up: Your muscles work and weight bear;
*   Elliptical machines are more rhythmic than stair climbers;
*   You can work the antagonistic muscles by exercising backwards. Continue to face the front of the machine, but move the legs in reverse mode as if running backwards.

Scientifically, the ground impact forces for elliptical training are equal to the ground impact of walking, or about one tenth the impact of running. Keep your motion rhythmic on a well-balanced machine and your wear and tear is essentially zero...provided you vary the settings on your machine. Just like in biking, you're placing strain upon your joints with every cycle of the legs: vary the amount of flexion at the ankle and knees, by spending two or three minutes at several crossramp levels. After warming up, you can give the calves and Achilles a thorough stretching and an eccentric workout by using a high incline for several minutes.

Note: Resistance and workload or workrate, and effort level are interchangeable phrases for elliptical machines. The same holds true for crossramp angle, incline, steepness or elevation level.

Buying an elliptical trainer?

Test drive them. Different models have different egg shapes to their ellipse. Some machines allow you to lengthen the stride and are more like an adapted ski machine. Other machines have an ellipse which is more like standing up on a bicycle for your sessions. Some machines allow arm movement with hand levers, giving you upper body exercise: If your arms are moving, you can maintain high heartrates with more modest effort from your leg muscles, which is ideal for rest days.

When buying, you'll also need to consider your desire for an attached heartrate monitor, how extensive the gym-style display is, their base length for steadiness and for excessive use of your house space, and the position of the handles (directly in front of your shoulders is ideal). Most runners will do fine with a $250 model to use for 20 minutes twice a week and get 200 workouts so it's a dollar 25 cents per session. According to Roy M. Wallock's article in the LA Times Health Section of April 14, 2,003, machines under $1,000 are apt to break. He reviewed 4 machines ranging in cost from $1,399 to $3,499. If you don't have a decent variety available to test, get information from the 4 companies Wallock reviewed, precor.com, lifefitness.com, schwinnfitness.com and visionfitness.com.

Belong to a gym? Their equipment will be renewed every year or two and they'll probably have a top of the line model. However, they may not suit your body type, and the commute may take the 30 minutes that you could actually use for the cross training.

Run at 10 minutes per mile? Because the elliptical machine does not mimic running perfectly, you'll need about 15 minutes to give the equivalent of a running mile. Because you'll probably be resting those big leg muscles a bit by holding onto the rails, you'll burn fewer calories than when running. Want the equivalent of a 4 mile run indoors because it's 20 below freezing or over 100 degrees outside? Elliptical for 15 minutes, run two decent paced miles on the treadmill and then finish with another 15 minutes on the elliptical machine.

Don't rely too much on a treadmills stated pace. They can be 20 seconds per mile off, the belts can slip and the speed change. 5,000 new ones were recalled by one company recently!

If you're doing page 191s fitness test at a set speed and you feel great despite your heartrate being 5 points higher, there's a good chance that you've been running 10 seconds per mile faster than thc trcadmill is telling you.

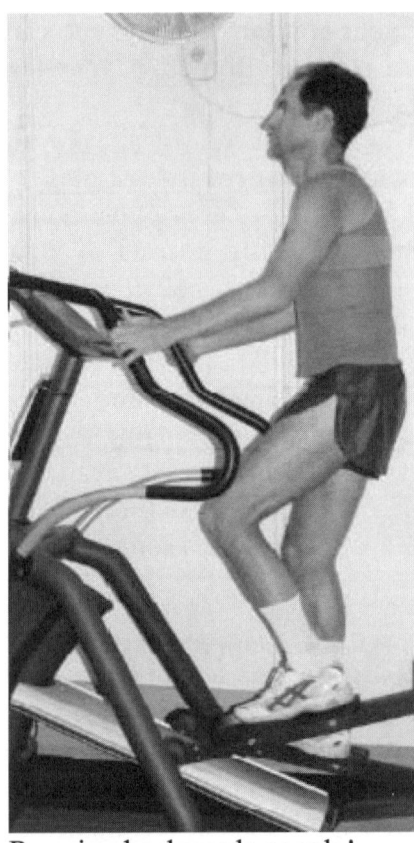

Runners with good balance can swing their arms instead of holding onto the supports. Got poor balance? Exercise at an intensity which allows you to stay on your feet with only a light low-stress grip on the side rails or handles. Our athlete on the left is holding on with three fingers to stop himself from falling backwards. He is moving his legs in a backwards motion.

Stand up straight with your belly pulled in. Ease into sessions with all parts of your body relaxed. Hold your head and shoulders up and no slouching.

Note that the right knee has about 15 degrees of flexion remaining at its straightest point. The calf is getting a nice stretch without impact.

Running backwards people!

Elliptical Training Sessions:

Done your 30 minutes of weight training? After all, it's the most important cross training! Then you're ready for the elliptical trainer. To avoid sudden changes in training, spend about 4 weeks getting used to the machine for 10 and building to 30 minutes at a time, using slight variations in resistance and incline to ease the tension on your knees and to get a fuller range of motion. After this 4 week preparation, during cross training sessions you can gently transition from weights to elliptical for five minutes, and try these:

<u>Session One:</u> Do 2 minutes going forward at a comfortable elevation and resistance while maintaining 90 strides (90 for each foot that is) per minute.

Then do 2 minutes with a backwards motion while facing the front of the machine. Use the same elevation, but because the hamstrings are supposed to be weaker than the thigh muscles, your workrate may need to be one or two notches lower.

Continue to alternate 2 minutes forward and backward, but increase the elevation one notch every 2 minutes until it becomes difficult to maintain with a relaxed motion. Then take it back one notch.

At 10 and 15 minutes, you might also increase the resistance a notch. Aim for your exercise intensity to reach anaerobic threshold at 20 minutes, and then maintain it for 5 more minutes.

For your warmdown, ease back on the elevation by one notch each minute while continuing to alternate the forward and backward motion every two minutes. Decrease the resistance also for the last two minutes.

Hint: When changing direction, ease to a stop over several seconds, adjust the resistance, and then recommence as if changing gently from a walk to easy running over several seconds.

Session Two: First 10 minutes as for session one, then:

Increase tempo to 100 strides per minute for one minute, ease back to 90 to cruise for one minute; change direction and repeat. Then, increase resistance or elevation by one notch for one minute at 100 strides. Rest at the original resistance, change direction and repeat.

Then use 2 followed by 3 additional notches of resistance or elevation to give yourself 8 intervals...4 in each direction.

Do a four-minute warmdown similar to session one.

Your goal: get up to 5K running intensity for the last 2 intervals without straining madly.

You can also use the pre-set interval sessions on the machine. Be sure they are at the appropriate intensity for your current days requirements and level of fatigue.

Cross training should complement your run training. You need to practice running at 5K effort or close to your VO2 maximum and at anaerobic threshold intensity for the psychomotor perfection of your running form. It is vital to be relaxed at these speeds. Generally, your longer interval sessions should be running.

If you do want to do a full session on the elliptical trainer as a substitute for running once every 2 to 3 weeks...increase the session to 45 minutes and stride elliptically for:

*   5 X 5 minutes at 85 % of max HR, and close to 100 cycles per minute for threshold training; switch direction after 3 minutes.
*   10 times 2 to 3 minutes at 90 to 98 % max HR, at just over 100 strides per minute for VO2 max training. Switch direction after each interval.
*   Most machines count the stride on both feet, so your speed days are at 200 of their strides, or 100 stride cycles.
*   Note: No arm movement means that your legs will be working about 10 percent harder to achieve 85 or 95 percent of max HR, so decrease target HR by 10 to 15 beats to save your legs.

You don't have to memorize these sessions. Just switch direction and elevation every 2 to 3 minutes.

There's little point in moving at greater than 100 stride cycles per minute. Even when running at 2-mile race pace you'll be doing less than 100. Increase resistance or incline a bit to get your heartrate up to 98 % of maximum to work on VO2 max.

Note: 75 percent of your training benefits come from the first half of your interval session. Restricting yourself to fifteen minutes of quality cross training is best for most runners. Save your legs to run productive interval sessions away from machines...though the treadmill has its uses.

Choice Three: The Bicycle

Ride indoors while watching an inspiring video, or outside with the stimulating elements...it depends on how stimulating those elements are. Lance Armstrong did a lot of running in his early days and still cross trains with running in winter. You can cross train on the bike. Bike riding studies show a 9 percent improvement in 10K race times, plus boosts in VO2 max, and no overstriding.

In bike riding, the effort is mostly on the thigh muscles, which will help your hill running ability...but without all those risks from ground impact, and therefore less muscle damage. When biking, the pressure on your joints and bones is less than when walking. In biking, the pressure is less than when merely standing. Cycling also loosens up your knee joints, making them less painful. Because you're working the thighs, biking complements pool running nicely. Point the toes down and you can give the calves a bit of work, but you'll still need to do some calf muscle exercises with weights or against your own body's resistance.

Want to exercise those hamstrings and calves better? Fit toe clips to your pedals so that you can pull up on each revolution. The natural tendency is to simply push down on the pedals, which means that the quads do all the work. You'll have to think about pulling the foot up on each revolution until it becomes second nature. You can also use cycling shoes of course, but unless you're riding greater than 50 miles, use the money to replace your running shoes more often. Use your old running shoes for biking.

Biking Regularly can:

* Increase your flexibility because you work running's antagonistic muscles.
* Decrease injuries;
* Improve cadence;
* Make your quadriceps stronger;
* Keep you fit while healing a tendon injury from running;
* If you have I-T band syndrome, you may want to use a recumbent bike, which reduces the flexion at the hip.

Chapter 16 stated that you could easily rest while biking downhill. Don't. Peddling at 90 to 100 revolutions with minimal resistance in easy gears, or maintaining modest legspeed while free-wheeling will bring nutrients into your muscle cells and get much of the lactic acid from the hill climb out of your muscles. When you start the serious effort again at the base of the hill, your muscle cells will be ready to work.

Inactively sitting on your butt for those downhills will leave your legs stiff, just like when you fail to warmdown after running a track session. You don't have to pedal hard like a professional biker. Maintaining your heartrate at 60 percent of your maximum will keep you in the training zone for the entire ride, instead of only on the flat and uphill.

Use the same rule when approaching red lights. Instead of maintaining hard effort and breaking severely...plan ahead. Coast or spin as you approach the light, and choose your exit gear for carefully getting through the junction.

The specificity rule mentioned before states that to run well you must train well with mostly running. You practice by running the exact pace you intend to race at, plus a few miles a bit faster to improve VO2 max, and plenty of miles a bit slower for endurance. Yet all three can be achieved with biking.

Biking lets you amass great training volume, but you need to incorporate some speed riding, and maintain speed running. You also need to practice the running push off from your toes to work the lower leg muscles, ankle and hamstrings. Maintain your fartlek, threshold pace and interval running, including a few downhill strides to stretch out the hamstrings and gluteal muscles.

Bikers have an easier time with hydration and other fuels. They can carry a ton of liquid on the bike and actually drink it. They can eat carbos with a little protein without being too concerned about it sloshing around in the stomach. An energy bar and 32 ounces of liquid in your belly is no problem when biking.

Standing on the bike for harsher workouts.

Having someone drive you back down the mountain after hour-long uphills will enable you to stand for most of your riding. Hill climbs allow you to achieve very high heartrates. Maintain a cadence of 90 to 100 to reduce the strain on the knees. Take an extra shirt to stay warm if you intend to coast back down with occasional spinning of your legs.

Alas, most people sit for the bulk of their bike riding. Sitting is more aerodynamic, but means the heartrate will be 10 percent lower than comparable running workouts.

Twenty to 30 mile rides at 70 percent of max HR twice a week does wonders for a runners endurance. Start by doing these rides instead of a 4 to 6 mile run for a few weeks, then gradually add back the easy run so that your total training volume has increased.

Prefer to substitute biking for running? It takes about three to four miles of biking to equal a single mile of running...if you're at appropriate intensity. I believe that biking for twice the time it takes to run a mile is equal to one mile of running. Current easy pace 7:30 per mile? Each quarter of an hour on a bike will give you a running mile equivalent. You may need to organize your life better to find the extra time required for biking instead of running, though it has great potential for commutes to work!

According to a study by Susan C. Gray Ph.D. and others, a few bursts before speed training will decrease the amount of lactic acid which you produce. That is also part of the reason you do striders before <u>running</u> any speed sessions. When you're comfortable with steady rides, add some threshold pace miles by doing 10 to 15 minutes pretty hard once, twice and then three times in one of your weekly rides. You should feel as if you'd be able to maintain that speed for 40 to 60 minutes. Heartrate should be 75-85 percent of max. Decrease your threshold running sessions the first few weeks while doing these bike intervals.

Working on VO2 max? Two to 5 minute efforts, at a pace you could handle for 15 to 20 minutes would work. Used to 8 x 800 meters at the track? Build toward 8 repeats of one mile on the bike. However, if your biking is in addition to a track session, doing 3 to 4 repeats will give a modest, yet VO2 max enhancing session. This bike session could be the day after your track session, or mere minutes afterwards. Practice good biking form and ride safely.

Four repeats give you about 75 percent of the training benefits of 8 repeats. Short sessions give a disproportionate reward for the effort put in: This half session is a runners best friend...big rewards from modest effort!

Want interval training with friends? Join a spinning class once or twice a week. It's indoors and you'll all be working at your own intensity. Before doing a spinning class however, you should be in good biking shape. You need to be bike fit before you do biking intervals. Set the resistance to your needs. The instructor may be inspirational, the music maybe fast, but keep the cadence below 110 and your intensity below 95 percent of maximum heartrate respectively in your early sessions. You need to be able to walk out of the club afterwards; you need to run 6 or 8 miles the next day.

Bike buying? Go cheap. This author recently purchased a mountain bike for $110. Helmet, shorts and sundries, and I was on the road for less than $175. Yes readers...the road. Wide tires with suspension front and back and 21 gears.

Like over 90 percent of mountain bikes, it will never experience a trail. This author on the other hand, does experience continuous high quality exercise for 50 to 95 minutes. It's slower than an 18 speed road bike, but it's safer at high heartrates because the speed is slower, and it's easier to view the road ahead.

Avoiding Bike Pains

Road Burn: Don't fall off your bike or crash into things! Plan ahead for traffic lights, stop signs and the actions of other animals. Break gently as a rule. Find a quiet dirt trail to practice fast stopping, and the art of getting one foot out of your toe clips in a timely manner. Wear safety clothing.

Backache: Distance from seat to handlebars should not stretch your body to discomfort. Ride with your elbows slightly bent and your back at no less than a 50-degree angle to the road. Arch and relax your back every 10 to 15 minutes to reduce muscle fatigue.

Knee pains: Adjust your seat height to get a slight bend at the knee when your foot is at its lowest point. Use easy gears at high cadence instead of straining with big cogs. As with running, keep the knees pointing straight ahead. Keep the patella tracking perfectly or your rides will give you chondromalacia. Push the saddle back if you need to.

Sore butt: Wear biking shorts for the extra cushioning. Some people say that squashing the artery and nerves for extended periods can compromise penis circulation. Ergonomic bike seats are built up each side to keep the perineal area and communication cords safe from most pressure. Other saddles have a triangular section cut out of the middle. Ride a bike with suspension front and back while avoiding rough trails and you'll further decrease your risk. Don't lean forward onto your perineum for extended periods. Being slim, healthy and fit are all aphrodisiacs.

Stiff neck: You've got to see where you're going. Move your head around frequently to reduce the neck strain. Mountain bike handlebars are great for runners. Unless you're riding with a fast group, you don't need to ride aerodynamically at 24 miles an hour (mph). You can sit up more, resisting the air at 21 mph. Your legs don't know and can't care.

Tingling hands: Caress rather than grip the handlebars. Change hand positions often. Stretch during breaks. Cruising handlebars are good for long rides.

Buy a bike to suit your build. The top tube, which runs from the seat to the handlebars, needs to be short if your body is short. Choose from road bikes to hybrids to mountain bikes depending on the size of tire width you feel comfortable with to the weight of bike you'll ride and lift into or onto a car. Health Magazine's April 2,003s issue shows bikes from: giant-bicycle.com, specialized.com and trekbikes.com in the $350 to $600 range. Check those sites and then test ride and get fitted at your local store.

Spending too much time away from your significant other? Check the tandem bikes at raleighusa.com for under $600. See runningbook.com for other sources.

Recumbent bikes are unlikely to come down in price until department stores sell them. Although you cannot stand on them, recumbents offer most cross-training benefits of traditional biking.
*   They give you a better view than racing bikes; you're always facing forward so you don't need to look up.
*   Large saddles which distribute your weight in a kinder manner. Some have a hammock style seat to distribute your weight on your butt and back.
*   Steering and breaking can be close to your hips or high like a Harley; either way, there's no pressure on your hands & arms.
*   There are now bike shops which sell only recumbents.
www.bikeroute.com/WhyBent.html has more info on recumbent biking or check: easyracers.com lightningbikes.com and visionrecumbent.com for bikes priced at $600 to $1,200.

Walking is good cross-training too.
You can walk for one to two minutes every 15 minutes during long runs while rehydrating, or you can walk 3 to 5 miles once or twice a week as cross training.

Studies on ground impact during exercise usually take your body weight as the base = 100. Walking scores about 115 compared to running's 250 to 300.

The problem, of course, is getting the heartrate up enough for runners to call it training. Wake up Mr. Paradox! Some of your exercise should be more for relaxation than training. You run easily at 60 to 80 percent of maximum heartrate for 4 to 6 miles for recovery and to maintain or achieve a solid base. Why not walk briskly, and with good form for those 40 to 60 minutes, and relax your way at 55 percent of maximum heartrate. It's possible to maintain 60 percent or more of max HR for 95 % of your walk according to some studies. You'll still burn over 100 calories per mile, and more if it's in deep sand. If walks are in addition to your running, you'll get fitter by building muscles and endurance, and perhaps by losing some weight.

Provided you use good walking technique, ground impact is not much more than when you're standing. Technique is essentially the same as for running, including:

Land with a bent knee;

Gently on the heel;

Roll through the ball of the foot;

Push off with your toes;

Swing the arms back and forward;

Keep your back straight and pull in your abdominals.

Note that race walkers use a straight leg at landing.

The main difference with walking is that there's always at least one foot on the ground. With running, both feet can be off the ground at the same time.

Want quality in your walking? Hills, treadmills, stadium steps, the stairs in high rise buildings or walking in the sand or with poles give limitless options for intervals of 2 to 10 minutes at 5K to 15K intensity. Use the elevator instead of walking back down the stairs. Keep the treadmill at zero gradient during recoveries, and you'll never suffer the ground impact of walking downhill. You can also enjoy your walking by avoiding intensity!

2,003 was the year of the 10,000 steps a day for health, and 2,004 is a free pedometer with almost every purchase to help you count those steps, but most people will still get the pedometer after driving to a fast food restaurant. Less than 40 percent of pedometers are accurate, so do a check with 500 steps at normal pace on asphalt, and other tests with 500 slower steps on carpet and on grass to check your pedometer.

Find ways to increase the amount of exercise that you do by walking to your lunch date, using the stairs, and parking at the farthest point from the shops at the mall.

Other options.

Cross-country skiing, inline skating or roller bladding are specialty sports which take practice and skill to achieve a decent aerobic workout. Research shows that it is easy to work at 90 percent of your maximum aerobic capacity during the novice stages of these sports: just like with running, you're inefficient at the beginning. With practice, your efficiency improves and your heartrate at a given speed will decrease. However, with experience you will be able to skate, ski or blade for a longer duration, and significantly increase your aerobic capacity with low impact forces.

The learning curve for a skiing machine is quite rapid. With small snowshoes, snow walking and running is an option for many. Hint: Even after the nastiest storms, there is usually running terrain somewhere close by.

Don't go overboard with these exercises. Many are so different to running that you're working a strange group of muscles: fine for cross-training because your running muscles can rest up. Don't strain the other muscles though.

The various forms of dance from jazz to hip-hop or salsa, or aerobic and step classes, with or without light dumb-bells are also a pleasant way to cross train, especially if the whether is nasty outside. Land gently though while keeping your heartrate in <u>your</u> range for a particular day. You can also do Interval aerobic classes for greater stimulation once you have the coordination.

Stair climbing machines are easy to use, build quadriceps power, but usually don't work the arms; stairs can also cause knee problems. However, rowing can correct a shoulder weakness.

<u>Rowing</u> is not close to making it into the top three aerobic exercises to best suit a runner's needs. This author is not even tempted to make it the forth choice, however, it does have a few things going for it:

* Rhythmic. You can keep going for a considerable time and stimulate the heart and lungs just like with running.
* It works the shoulders. Much less than with swimming, but more than during running.
* You can enjoy the scenery on the river or lake, though you're more likely to be indoors, on a machine.

* It works your torso or to use the 2,003 in phrase, it works your core muscles; it also works most of the leg muscles.

Every time you push your legs straight in rowing you do a leg-press. The leg-press, lunge and squats are ideal weight training exercises because you work the quadriceps, hamstring and gluteal or buttock muscles. In rowing, you do a leg-press 30 to 40 times every minute for your 10 to 20 minute session. You work the shoulder and arm muscles while giving abdominals and back a goodly bit of work to do. Whether on a rowing machine before your elliptical session or out on the water, admiring where you've been as you row backward, here's how to row.

* In the first part of the drive, push out with your legs while moving your back from its arched position toward sitting up straight. Pull back with your arms and at full extension of the legs, don't stretch your back out as you lean back just a bit.
* Don't lock out. Keep a few degrees of extension in reserve at your elbows and knees.
* Pull yourself back to the front of the machine to work the hamstrings. Knees should be in line with your ankles and in line with your hips. Don't bow them in or out. Flex your knees to your tolerance, which may not be the front of the machine.
* Keep your shoulders back; avoid the tendency to round them forward when extending the arms forward.

US Rowing Association (800) 314-4769 or www.usrowing.org
Kayaking and canoeing are too focused on the arms for runners.

Your lungs, heart and the rest of your circulatory system are not too worried about which type of (mainly) aerobic exercise you do. Your mind and your racing ability do need fun exercise and specific exercise respectively. If you find a mix of exercise which is enjoyable, and do about 20 % of it fairly intensely, you'll do it often enough to race well. However, as stated before, running must dominate.

Stride Frequency.

Whether walking or running, the best stride rate is 90 to 95 steps with each foot per minute for most people. Long strides can cause great impact with each step, slowing you down and sending vibrations up your body, which increase injury risk.

Fortunately, there's a near perfect correlation between stride rate and stride length. Increase your cadence to greater than 90 per minute and your stride length is forced to shorten. Practice rapid and short strides on grass twice a week and up short hills to reduce your over-striding risk.

Practice rapid cadence at a rhythmic 100 per minute during cycling and elliptical training also, to help increase your stride rate.

The ability to run fast comes from leg muscle strength and oxygen uptake. Long steady runs, appropriately paced speed sessions, plus balanced cross training gives you the raw materials to run fast.

The table on page 188 shows the approximate amount of training time for a 10 minute mile person to get the equivalent of one mile of running from cross training, plus the percentage of training time for the rest of you to work out your cross training needs.

If you buy a piece of exercise equipment for cross training, use it on at least one set day every week. If you're not using it a second time each week on an ad hoc basis after three months, set another "must do" session each week.

Elliptical machines and outdoor bike buying has been covered. You can consider an exercise bike to use as a warm up before going out into the cold, or for warming down with liquids in front of you and a fan on hot days. While you should do most of your exercise outside for a better life and an energy boost from the elements, some days you'll want to stay indoors for the entire session.

In early 2,004 I needed to test a pair of running shoes at a store and was a little disappointed when the sales person plugged in a $400 treadmill instead of its $3,000 neighbor. Much to my surprise, the $400 version gave a very nice ride at 6:30 mile pace and caused me to get two pairs of shoes.

There is probably enough exercise equipment collecting dust under beds and in cellars in the U.S. to equip thousands of gyms. Set up your stuff so that it's easy to use on nasty weather days, or no baby sitter days, or must watch game 5 of the play-offs day, or just don't feel like running outside days.

For the 10 minute miler;   The rest of you;

Activity	Time to equal one mile	percent	comment
Running	10 minutes or	100 %	a mile is a mile
Weights	30 mins	300 %	(See note one below)
Pool runs	10 mins	100 %	the perfect match
Elliptical	15 mins	150 %	very close match
Biking	20 mins	200 %	decent match
Rowing	21 mins	210 %	good strength session
Ski machine	21 mins	210 %	useful aerobic session
Snow shoe running	15 mins	150 %	if you're at 75 % of max HR

Roller bladding, cross-country skiing, skating, or snow shoe walking,   31 mins   310 %   (See note two below)

Note One: Weights are still the most important cross training. True, a 30 minute session will only give you one mile of running, but it takes time to set up machines; unless you do circuit training type weights, your heartrate will rarely go above 100.

Note Two: Too specialized and unlikely to be continuous at appropriate heartrates. Factor in the downhills and socializing and they are unlikely to do much for your running, though they are fun and burn calories, which could improve your running.

Good cross-country skiers can maintain high heartrates for long periods without injury. In fact, Norway's two greats of the 1980s at the marathon, Kristiansen and Waitz, trained copiously with cross-country skiing. They were also pretty fast at the 5K. Skiing is a great way to get outside exercise during harsh winters. Novice skiers need to be patient while learning the skills, yet their heartrates will also be high, but mainly due to inefficiency on skis.

An eight minute per mile person can match his 5 mile easy run in 40 minutes with sessions of 40 x 150 % for 60 minutes on the elliptical machine, or 40 x 200 % for 80 minutes of biking, etc.

However, if he follows the advice of the last 46 pages, he will weight train for 36 minutes, then elliptical for 42 minutes. His second session of weights later in the week would be followed by pool running for 28 minutes.

Chapter Eighteen

Concluding Tips

This and a couple other chapters share a common heritage in <u>Best Half-Marathons</u>. As these tips are fundamental to all runners, and most of you will not be running half-marathons, please enjoy these extra tips. Some of these tips could have been in Chapter Two and many of them restate earlier themes. You all have different needs for your training book, so use or merely peruse.

The most important exercise session is the one following your races. Keep your motivation high for fitness exercise and for running by knowing that you will race again in 3 to 6 weeks.

In the meantime, eight to 24 hours post race, walk a couple of miles and take another warm shower. Session two could be another walk or an easy 3 mile run. Session three might be a one-hour bike ride if you were used to riding before the race. Then ease back up to 4-6 mile runs and gentle striders.

<u>Doing any session for the first time?</u> Don't do much.

First run in 5 years? Walk for 5 minutes to warm up, start your run very slowly and ease to a walk after one hundred yards or meters. Alternate walking with short bouts of running for a mile. Shower and stretch gently.

<u>First speed session?</u> After a mile of easy running and your

stretches, run half a mile of repeats at the appropriate pace. Run 30 seconds slower than 5K pace to improve your endurance and anaerobic threshold; do this once a week and add a quarter mile each week. A couple of months later, add a separate session at 5K pace each week to improve your running economy and oxygen uptake or VO2 maximum. Do not sprint.

Start every session gently. Aiming for 5 miles in 50 minutes, which you know will be 75 percent of your maximum heartrate? Run the first mile in 10:30, pick up your pace ending the fourth mile at 9:45 pace and back off to 10 minute pace to finish. Walk 200 meters before and after the run.

Speed sessions too. Run the first two repeats or the first half mile a bit slower than goal pace for the session. Example: Want 8 x 400 meters in 90 seconds because you race the 5K in 19 minutes. Run two repeats each at 92, 90 and 88 before showing your self control with 90s to finish and see Chapter 11.

Want a change of pace come race day? Practice it in training. Looking for six-minute miles and a surge? Run 800 meters with the first lap in 92 seconds and the second lap in 88. The "differential" is 16 seconds per mile. Keep good running form for the second lap of each repetition.

Monthly races will motivate you, giving you a reason to rest for a week. Rest means doing 60 % of your average weekly mileage. Races make your game more sociable and give an incentive to run 5 times 800 meters at 10 seconds per mile faster than your last 5K race for one session every three weeks. The other two weeks you'll do longer repeats.

Take long rests in speed training at first. Those 800s may need a four-minute rest the first time. Edge the recovery down by 30 seconds per month to reach 90 or 60 seconds.

Feeling unmotivated for days at a time? Dissatisfied with your running and performances? Heartrate elevated when you wake up? Sleeping poorly, with achy muscles and loss of weight? You could have been overtraining. Decrease mileage for a few days or weeks if necessary.

<u>Catabolism</u> is the breaking down of body structures, especially the muscles, due to doing too much. The sympathetic nervous system is sympathetic to your desire to be active for 18 or 19 hours per day, to eating negligible amounts of nutritious food, to your impending divorce or troubled child, to your nasty boss, to the "can't decide where I'm going" stock market, and to your reckless 4 miles of repeats at the track.

Watch for increased resting heartrate, weight loss or gain, poor training or sleep or decreased interest in your favorite activities as an indication to rest up, including decent amounts of sleep.

To avoid overtraining, set realistic goals which you can achieve based on current fitness, instead of based on your dream fitness level. Run a few striders of 200 meters at 5K pace twice a week for the joy of it instead of training for a race. Elsewhere, slow down to 65 percent of maximum heartrate for your running. Cross train gently for recreation and a social life and to see different scenery during exercise sessions.

Decrease the risk of overtraining by making only small changes to your training. Add a mile or 10 minutes of running once a week, or increase your exercise duration for the entire week by 10 percent for up to three weeks, but then consolidate to let your muscles and circulatory system catch up to the demands.

Adding speed running? Run at the right intensities as shown in earlier chapters. Match every speed run with a steady paced run.

Overtraining Fitness Test.

The above are useful signs to spot fatigue from overtraining, and that you need to take a few days or weeks of recovery exercise, but a regular, easily achieved pace run is an excellent back-up.

A pace run is a fitness test not a time trial. You will run a modest distance such as 2 miles, but at a set, easily achieved speed. You'll use the same speed for an entire year or more. You can do it every 2 weeks or so and be fresh enough afterwards that unless the test showed overtraining, you can finish your days exercise with some gentle speed running at 5K pace.

45 seconds slower than 5K speed is a good choice for your pace run. It's slower than anaerobic threshold, and at 2 miles it's also shorter than your tempo sessions.

You will monitor your heartrate during these fitness test runs. A heartrate monitor lets you check every quarter of a mile and you can make a mental note of your heartrate. You should reach your usual test pace heartrate at about the one mile point, and because you focus on running economically, it should stay at that level for all 4 checks leading to 2 miles.

An increased heartrate at your regular pace indicates overtraining, so jog for 5 to 10 minutes and plan several easy days. Treadmills allow you to repeat the same conditions every time, and almost guarantee even pace (but see page 175). A track also makes checking your splits and heartrate easier. You can also use a flat road or path, check your heartrate at definite points, and rely on your pacing skills.

Drafting (running behind another person) is legal and saves your energy. Drafting can be worth 15 seconds in a 5K. Other runners must be at your desired pace. Don't run fast in order to stay with a group. Once the pace drops, it's your turn to set the pace, so expect others to draft behind you. Don't weave. You could soon be drafting off of them again!

Practice drafting during speed sessions as you alternate being the lead person. There is an art to staying close without tripping each other up. Stay far enough away from the person to run relaxed and stress free, but close enough to benefit from the drafting. Some people never get it, but they can still benefit mentally while running 5 meters behind the group because they will not have to think about or set the pace. They merely cruise at the groups speed.

Don't race your friends. You may run 6 miles with him every Sunday, but his 5K speed can be 30 seconds per mile faster. Race the first mile with him and you're destined to pain and slowing in the other 2.1 miles. Start races at realistic pace for you.

Don't race your friend in training either. While it's nice to be more compatible, you can train with someone 2 minutes faster than you are at the 5K. While she runs long repeats at her anaerobic threshold, you can run short ones at your 5K pace by doing the first and last lap of her mile repeats.

Smaller 5K disparity? Persuade the faster runners to start 2 to 4 seconds after you do, so that they can chase you down. If all of you run at appropriate speed, you should reach the finish of the repeat at the same moment.

If a friend runs with you to start a fitness program,
he or she must run very slowly at your pace to ensure that you do not ache afterwards. This will be your friends rest day, when she or he needs no training benefit from the exercise. At some distant date, you may cruise effortlessly by each others side for several miles, but in the early days it's walking and easy running to help you learn how to get into shape.

Use a double knot to tie your training and racing shoes, but
don't suffocate your feet. Tuck the ends of your laces in. Lightweight or performance training shoes are best for most races. They give you more protection than racing flats.

Weight train and cross train until the penultimate week before a big race.
Don't increase the number of repeats, or the weight lifted in the last month. Instead, decrease repeats from 12 to 10 and then to 8 over the last three weeks to taper. Weight train at 4 or 5 day intervals instead of 3 days. Lift only 75 percent of your usual amount seven days pre-race as your last session.

Wear lightweight sweats to stay warm during and after
your warmup. Stretch gently before races and speed running. Then wear the smallest amount of clothing for the conditions.

You cannot convert fat to muscle. They are two distinct
body tissues. Exercise regularly and with modest increases in duration or resistance and you'll build larger and stronger muscle fibers. If you exercise more than you used too while consuming the same number of calories, you'll lose weight...generally via fat cells decreasing in size.

You cannot body sculpt. You cannot decide which part
of your body the fat will leave from. The leg press won't improve

the shape of your buns until you've burned off sufficient fat for those underlying muscles to show through a thinner fat layer.

The most important nutrient is water. Focus on the

water, not what form it comes in. Cold water is absorbed just as fast, and unless you're training for over two hours, water is generally all you need. Bonking in a 5K is due to lack of fitness, not lack of fuel in your body.

You sweat out very little salt. Pleasant tasting food will give you all the replacement you need...provided you include decent amounts of fruit and vegetables.

While studies have shown a 37 percent increase in peak performance when downing 200 calories with liquid, AKA a sports drink instead of water; the studies are usually based on:

o Cyclists, who can actually consume 32 ounces of liquid while moving at 90 percent of maximum heartrate;

o Sprinting to exhaustion at very high intensity at the end of a 60 or 90 minute session which was at fairly high intensity.

You, on the other hand are only running a 5K, and should start a moderate intensity surge at the 2-mile point to run a great race.

Breakthroughs in life usually come from moderate amounts

of effort on a consistent basis. Overnight success takes years of preparation! Cram in extra runs or more speed running in the days pre-race and you'll bomb in the race. A series of runs over many months, plus rest, sets you up for improved fitness and faster races.

Don't ever "hammer" your workout. Enjoy your

exercise. It annoys me to read experts who say you need to get sufficient rest on your easy days so that you can hammer your hard workouts. Work is something you do for 8 to 12 hours a day, but you don't go all out in the first minute...unless you want to be asleep with exhaustion in half an hour. True, your easy running days should be less intense than your faster training days. But, you should never be hammering your harsher exercise days.

* You run long efforts at 30 seconds per mile slower than 5K pace to improve your anaerobic threshold;

* You run at 5K to 2 mile pace for one to six minute repeats to improve your VO2 max and running efficiency;

* You run hills for strength, but mostly at 3K intensity.
* Run at 90 to 95 strides for each foot per minute to avoid over-striding, which increases injury risk. Increase stride rate or cadence and you'll decrease your stride length, and run faster.

True, the last couple of repeats will usually feel harder than the first few, but you should not feel hammered because you will have spent weeks building up to these sessions. You should feel as if you could do more repeats, but you warmdown instead.

Mix in rest days and long runs every 7 to 10 days, and your two quality sessions each week should not give you sore muscles which take days to recover from. They will gradually prepare you for higher levels of health and fitness, or great races.

Still looking for an illusive personal record? Get a
friend to pace you accurately for key Intervals of long repeats, and pace you on a flat 5K course with minimal turns at 50 to 60 degrees Fahrenheit: Rest up properly, and a PR is highly probable.

Fatigue will catch up with you. Your quads and calves
especially do an eccentric muscle contraction every time you land, thus storing some of the incoming energy. After a few miles your eccentric abilities decrease and you'll:

* Spend more time actually on your feet;
* The braking and storing of elastic energy takes longer;
* Stride rate decreases, so you slow down.

Your body compensates by bending a bit more at the knees, unfortunately this is less efficient. Our nervous system also recruits the last of our muscle fibers to keep us going at our desired pace. You can help this recruitment by:

1. Running more miles per week, including,
2. Hill training;
3. Anaerobic threshold running;
4. Short Intervals at 5K to 3K pace, as preparation for;
5. Long Intervals at 3K to 10K pace, so that you learn to;
6. Take shorter strides to delay fatigue;
7. And run upright and tall with a minimal forward lean.

8. Doing regular plyometric exercises.

If you keep going with muscles and tendons unable to stretch during the stretch-shortening or eccentric cycle, you risk injury.

Mythical Second Wind.

Start at the right pace in training runs and races and you will not get a second wind. When you start too fast, your cardiovascular system gets a shock and your heartrate goes very high. After 5 to 15 minutes, your blood is mainly in the running muscles and your heartrate settles down as you find an economical running rhythm, plus the chemicals contributing to a runner's high begin to hit your brain. You appear to get a second wind.

When you're doing a fairly tough session think about its *purpose* as you gobble up the planet at faster than average speed.

Plyometrics for leg strength.

Page 101 mentioned bounding as part of the hill training chapter. For the first six months of your running life, bounding is the only plyometric exercise you need in order to add explosive power to your muscles.

Plyometrics improve running economy by decreasing the amount of oxygen you consume per mile of running. So:

In your second six months, add skipping with or without a rope. Shifting forward with rapid 6 inch strides, with a running type movement for your arms is probably best, and increases your calf muscles' resistance to fatigue from their eccentric contractions. 100 skips give you a 50 feet starting goal. After walking for 20 to 30 seconds, do another 100, then finish off your run.

As usual you've started gently, and should not get calf cramps that night. Three days later, do 3 x 100 skips, and gradually move it up to 4 or 5 times 200 skips over the course of 10 sessions. Twice a week should suffice because you'll also do some bounding exercises on these days. Focus on the ankles flicking through nicely and whipping off the end of your toes and after six months you'll be ready to add:

Hopping: Start with your feet together and on soft grass. Jump up about 6 inches and forward 18 inches while keeping your feet together. Pretty tame you'll think, so do another nine while learning to maintain balance. Walk for 30 seconds and then do a set of 15 jumps, then skipping and bounding.

Three days later you can hop a few inches farther per hop or higher but land softly or you'll set yourself up for shin splints or worse. Soft sand at the beach works nicely for hopping and your bounding. After three months you'll be up to full height and distance for 10 to 20 hops and 5 or 6 sets. You can then incorporate some single leg hops for half of the sets, and consider:

The split-squat jump, which you do from a lunge position. Jump forward and upward propelling yourself with one leg at a time and landing ready for your next lunge with the opposite leg pushing off. You can also do the frog hop, which starts from a squat position. Jump up and forward and absorb the ground impact like a frog does with flexed limbs. Prepare for these plyometric exercises with lunges in the weight room and with slow walking lunges.

According to a study from Ohio State University, you get the same benefits from doing plyometrics in water. Try shallow rivers, the beach and the pool.

Overtraining and Delayed Onset Muscle Soreness

or DOMS, are somewhat different. Overtraining usually relates to an entire exercise program in which you wear yourself down until illness of injury prevents you from exercising. The fitness test on page 191 and other tips in this chapter, plus a graduated program should keep you away from overtraining.

The severe muscle aches from DOMS occurs from 24 to 96 hours after a particularly harsh session, peaking at 48 to 72 hours. It can be part of a plan such as 4 x one mile at 5K pace as a challenge and fitness test about three weeks before a 10K race.

DOMS usually occurs due to unplanned mistakes like doing 15 minutes of hill repeats because you just read an article on it. Avoid sudden changes. If you make a mistake, take 4 to 6 easy days to recover because another hard run will strain those achy muscles.

Want to take your 5K running to the next level?

Concentrate on the 10K with *10K & 5K Running, Training & Racing*. Improve your 10K by one minute, then come back and use that strength to take 30 seconds off your 5K time.

Appendix One

Over 20 Health Benefits

Of Regular Exercise

Here is a summary of the health benefits of regular exercise...expanded from "Why Exercise" at www.runningbook.com

Exchange running for walking if you like. Running gives the same health benefits when done at appropriate intensity.

Injections of Human Growth Hormone turn back your body clock by decades. Human Growth Hormone:

* Increases muscle mass,
* Strengthens bones,
* Increases stamina and vitality,
* Increases cardiac output and energy,
* Decreases blood pressure,
* Improves cholesterol profile,
* Improves sleep and vision,
* Improves psychological well-being and memory,
* Strengthens the immune system, and,
* Increases fertility, sexual desire and performance.

But you don't need injections to get Human Growth Hormone. You just need regular doses of exercise which will stimulate your body to produce its own Human Growth Hormone. Exercise is also much cheaper than hormonal injections and much less painful. In fact, provided you do it at the right intensity, there is no pain at all with exercise.

While most of the following benefits are based on 40 to 60 minutes of exercise per day, numerous studies show significant health benefits with just 10 minute sessions, done three times per day. Doing some sit-ups, press-ups and dumb-bell work before your morning shower, walking 15 flights of stairs during your lunch-break and taking the dog for a short but brisk walk will give the same health benefits as a 30 minute run.

When your goal is improved oxygen uptake or VO2 max to run a 5K you'll have to keep the focus on 30 minutes or more per session.

Burning calories your main goal? Longish sessions of aerobic exercise wins, but you also need to modify calorie intake for long term success.

1. Walking or running extends your life.

Cardiovascular disease, which encompasses the heart and the blood vessels, is the leading cause of death nationwide, surpassing one million kills per year. Coronary heart disease alone causes close to half a million deaths in the United States *every* year. Walking reduces heart attack risk and helps you to lose weight. Running reduces inflammation inside your blood vessels, which further reduces the risk of heart disease.

90 percent of people who have heart attacks have at least one risk factor such as high cholesterol, hypertension, diabetes, smoking or inactivity. Inactivity doubles your risk of heart disease. People who can run a mile in under 7:30 are at low heart attack risk.

According to a 12-year study, (New England Journal of Medicine, Jan 8, 1998), retired men who walked more than 2 miles a day lived longer than those who walked less than a mile a day. Only 23.8% of the 14 mile plus per week group died, whereas 40.5% from the lower mileage group died during the study period.

Women benefit too: 3 hours per week of brisk walking decreased heart attacks by nearly 40 percent. 5 hours per week ladies cut their risk by over 50 percent. (According to an analysis of the 72,488 women in the Nurses Health Study). The bonus 10 percent probably comes from weight loss as most cardiovascular benefits occur at 20 to 30 minutes per day.

Try not to give yourself a heart attack in your first few exercise sessions. Start gently and stay hydrated. Whether at rest or during exercise, if you feel fullness, tightness, pressure or pain in the center of your chest; if the pain spreads to your shoulders, neck, back or arms; if you break into a cold sweat, feel lightheaded or short of breath: call 911 to get a diagnosis.

Although this book recommends exercising at 60 percent of maximum heartrate in the early days, for the full cardiovascular benefits you'll eventually need some exercise at 70 to 85 percent of max. Chapters 6 to 8 will be your main area of interest.

A multivitamin each day can reduce your chance of a heart attack by 33 percent. Low-dose aspirin also reduced heart attack risk by 32 percent. Moderate consumption of red wine (a glass a day) or one 12 ounce beer have been shown to improve circulation, but so has black tea. Four cups of tea give enough antioxidants or flavonoids to help the endothelium or inner lining of blood vessels. Healthy endothelium expands as the blood flow increases: owners of healthy endothelium are less likely to get heart disease. You still need to eat your veggies and fruit and you still need to exercise. Apples and apple juice contains tannins, which have anti-adhesion properties, also reducing the risk of circulatory diseases.

Eat a variety of fruit and vegetables to get all the nutrients required for good health. High fiber foods reduce your heart disease risk and hot tea's flavonoids decrease heart attacks. Nuts contain monounsaturated fat, omega-3s, phytochemicals, magnesium and the antioxidant vitamin E, all of which decrease heart disease risk. Nuts also keep you feeling full longer, which can help your weight loss goals. Don't eat the flavored varieties with trans fats (avoid if partially hydrogenated is on the label).

Omega-3 fats protect the heart and blood vessels from damage, so consume oily fish such as salmon, tuna and cod, or flaxseed (and its oil), pumpkin seeds, arugula, kale, mustard greens and nuts. The prostaglandins made from omega-3s tell blood vessels to dilate, keep your blood fluid, and reduce inflammation, which is good for your muscles and your brain.

Magnesium is one of the most likely nutrients to be needed IV if you're in hospital with heart trouble. Decrease heart disease risk by 45 percent with 400 milligrams per day from bananas (32 mg), broccoli (33), Salmon (42 in 4 ounces), milk (27 per cup), peanut butter (28 per tablespoon) and other nuts in their purest state.

And get off the sofa to exercise. Always warmdown at the end of runs. Slow down significantly for 5 minutes, and also walk for a few hundred yards. Hydrate to prevent blood clots though.

Peripheral arterial disease (PAD) can also be improved with steady exercise. Walk or jog through the leg cramps to a small degree of muscle pain and for a few minutes more, and then ease off. Do this several times to improve your walking and jogging endurance as the blood vessels get better at handling modest exercise. Non-exercisers are more likely to need surgery for their Peripheral arterial disease.

The two hour per week exercising man has a 60 percent less risk of a heart attack. It takes a mere 17 minutes per day and you can do different aerobic or weight training sessions every day. Get a heart disease risk assessment at

www.hin.nhlbi.nih.gov/atpiii/calculator.asp

americanheart.org includes many walking and running events. But runners are not immune from heart attacks.

Warnings of heart trouble in the near future include increased fatigue, shortness of breath, anxiety or feeling of impending doom, or indigestion.

Long runs result in minor muscle breakdown, which gives off chemical signs similar to the muscle damage of a heart attack. It's probably not your heart muscle which is damaged. It's simply the wear and tear from a pleasant, yet long run. When the ER doctor checks your creatine kinase-MB or other indicator of muscle damage, remind him or her about your most recent harsh training. Your EKG is also likely to suggest heart trouble due to PVCs and slow rate. A competent specialist will spot the athletic nature of your rhythm...especially if you let her know you're an athlete. Get a C-reactive protein or CRP test for another heart health guide, this time it's related to inflammation.

Eat some nice meals with normal protein amounts and your muscles will be stronger within a few days.

Post exercise collapse is a problem if you come to a sudden stop during harsh running, up hill running, long runs or after a race. It is probably due to a sudden drop in blood pressure as the blood pools in your leg muscles, combined with a dilation of your blood vessels further depriving your heart of its blood. Less blood gets back up to your heart and your poor brain gets even less than it did when you were cruising at race pace. You fall to the ground.

If you feel faint, get onto the ground in a controlled manner, stretch your legs out and lay your head down. Unless you know that you're dehydrated, only take a few <u>sips</u> of liquid. Poor some water over your head and put your feet up higher than your head if possible and do some ankle flexing to pump the blood out.

<u>Symptoms of Heartburn</u>, courtesy of your stomach contents include: Sharp burning sensation below the ribs especially after or soon after eating, and can be decreased with antacids. You probably will not be in a cold sweat.

Use these simple guidelines to decrease your heartburn:

* Eat minimal protein in the 2 hours before exercise because it slows the emptying from your stomach.
* Eat minimal fat in the 2 hours before exercise because it stimulates the release of bile into your stomach.
* Keep fiber to a minimal for that last pre-run meal.
* Which leaves the trusty carbohydrates. Monitor intake of citrus fruits, drinks with more than 6 percent sugar, or containing caffeine.
* Spicy or fatty food can affect you for 6 hours or more.
* Stay hydrated before and during runs. Liquid slushing around in your stomach for over 15 minutes? There's probably too much sugar in it, so drink some water.
* Control your race anxiety or your stomachs emptying will be delayed. Can't control yourself with relaxation techniques? Allow an extra hour after your last snack before running.

2. Walking lowers Stroke risk.

Stroke or cerebrovascular accident (CVA) is the third biggest killer, taking about 167,000 American lives per year, but it's no accident. Note: Factor in vascular diseases, and Diabetes would be the third biggest killer.

Burning Calories Cuts Your Stroke Risk. Burn 1,000 calories a week with exercise, such as walking briskly for 30 minutes, five days a week, can lower your stroke risk by 24%. According to a study of more than 11,000 men (Stroke, Oct 1998), exercise to the tune of 2,000 calories a week and you'll cut your stroke risk by nearly half.

Your exercise need only be moderately intensive. Brisk walking, dancing, bicycling or running are ideal.

According to a study of nearly 16,000 men and women (American Heart Association Scientific Sessions, Dallas, Nov 1998), exercise at work also decreases stroke risk. Those who were most active, such as walking, standing, or lifting heavy loads the most, had half the stroke risk.

Exercise may protect against stroke by modifying risk factors such as high blood pressure, body weight and potential for blood clots: Exercise also improves your brains circulation due to less plaque being laid down in the vital arteries.

Stroke is also called a cerebral vascular accident or CVA, but if you can reduce your CVA risk by half with simple exercise, a CVA is no accident: a CVA is the result of neglecting to exercise.

Stroke is the leading cause of disability in the United States. According to a 13 year study of the 50-plus Running Club at Stanford University, running decreased disability and death.

Decent potassium intake reduces the risk of hypertension and stroke. To get your 2,000 mgs per day of potassium, make friends with watermelon, cantaloupe, bananas, apricots, potatoes, milk and citrus fruits. Sadly, food products are not required to list their potassium content.

Take in 2 to 3 times the RDA for vitamin E or 133 mgs of vitamin C to lower your stroke risk by 20 and 30 percent. See *301 Nutrition Tips* for the best sources for these antioxidants.

People with healthy teeth and gums are less likely to have strokes or heart trouble. Regular flossing reduces blood vessel damage from the bacteria associated with periodontal disease.

Poor circulation is the first and third leading cause of death, but what is the second biggest murderer? Smoking and second hand smoke is the second leading cause of death in the United States. Smokers are 20 times more likely to get lung cancer and even more likely to die from the cancer. Smokers are 40 percent more likely to get colorectal cancer. Smoker's cancers are usually more advanced at diagnosis; smokers are more likely to be unhealthy and are more likely to die soon after diagnosis. Avoid smokers to extend your life. Exercise regularly to enjoy your life.

While the first two reasons for exercising are probably the most significant in terms of potential lifespan increase, the remaining 20 plus reasons to exercise are not in any particular order. We all have a special reason or need to exercise. Your friends reason may be different to yours, though both of you will be better off for exercising regularly.

3. Save your gallbladder.

According to a study at the Harvard School of Public Health, women who exercise two to three hours per week cut their gall-bladder surgery by 31 percent compared with women who don't exercise at all. Men who exercise 30 minutes per day on 5 days per week reduce their risk by 34 percent.

Over 300,000 women have their gallbladders taken out each year. Obesity and rapid weight loss increase the risk of gallstones. Lose weight slowly and keep it off!

As 80 percent of the gallstones in this country are solid choles-terol, lowering your cholesterol level should help avoid the gall-bladder cut.

Women with desk jobs are more likely to need their gallbladders removed...especially if they are also inactive in their recreational habits.

As with prostate and most other surgeries, regular exercise and being active decreases surgery complications.

Adequate intake of vitamin C also improves your healing capacity from surgery and recovery from exercise, while decreasing your risk of gallbladder problems.

My fellows in the United Kingdom showed up to a 60 percent decrease in gallstones with an hour per day of exercise. Hint: some days it will be your gardening or house cleaning. Five days a week it will include your running.

4. Listen! Exercise decreases blood pressure.

Hypertension is said to be the silent disease because it produces few outward symptoms, yet it doubles your risk of heart attack and is the leading risk factor for stroke and other heart diseases. One in four Yankees is hypertensive, which means a blood pressure of 140/90 or above. Millions more are pre-hypertensive with a systolic pressure of 121 to 139 and or a diastolic pressure of 71 to 89. The higher your blood pressure is, the higher your risk of circulatory diseases. Use regular exercise and healthful eating such as the DASH diet to reduce your hearts workload and lower your risk from a slew of hypertension related ailments.

No time for exercise? According to researchers at McMaster University in Hamilton, Ontario, 10 minutes of aerobic exercise will decrease blood pressure. Twenty to 30 minutes would be better, but surely you can find 10 minutes to preserve your life. Morticians can't preserve your life; regular, modest amounts of exercise will delay your visit to the mortician!

Losing a mere 10 pounds with exercise and a balanced, low fat and complex carbo diet will reduce your blood pressure; reduce your sodium intake slightly and you'll have taken three key steps. Inspired by the overweight, non-sweating (that is inactive) majority, the National Academy of Sciences lowered the recommended daily intake of sodium to 1,500 mgs. As you lose close to this amount per hour of running, don't overly restrict salt intake, but do keep processed food intake to a minimum, and avoid the salt shaker except on really hot days and humid days…though only if you left your air conditioned hovel.

Aim for 1.5 times as much potassium as sodium intake to decrease systolic blood pressure by 2.4 points, and therefore heart disease risk by 4.8 percent. Watch for excessive potassium intake if you're enamored by huge amounts of cantaloupe, apricots, peaches, oranges and bananas. Eat good fruits and everything else in moderation.

Wine, grapes and grape juice are also beneficial to hypertensives. In a study presented at the Experimental Biology meeting in San Diego in April, 2003, 12 ounces of grape juice per day had decreased the participant's systolic and diastolic pressure by nearly 6 points. Grapes improve the flexibility of artery walls, and this significant drop in blood pressure will decrease stroke risk by over 14 percent and heart disease by over 9 percent. Steal the calories your grape juice provides from your excess bread or other juices to ensure that you don't put on weight! Grape's anti-oxidants will soon be available in pill form to save you calories. Apples and blueberries also help your blood pressure, so rotate your fruit consumption.

You can drop your blood pressure just as much by eating ½ a cup of low-salt, roasted soy nuts. Unsaturated oils also help hypertensives. 35 grams of sesame oil per day for 60 days dropped a groups pressure from an average of 166/101 to a very respectable 134/85. Don't substitute for canola or olive oil. Use sesame oil instead of some of the rest of your saturated fat.

Weight training 3 times for 45 minutes per week dropped systolic pressure by 9 points and diastolic pressure by 8 points. Having a pet decreases pressure by 8 points. More tips on page 213, but men who get their blood pressure back to normal are likely to have 25 percent more sex, secondary to better blood flow and firmer erections.

5. Exercise decreases side effects of diabetes.

Exercise can control adult onset or Type II diabetes. Type II diabetes messes with the way your body utilizes sugar. In type II diabetes, either your body makes insufficient insulin, or your body can't use the insulin very well; you develop insulin resistance. With either scenario, your body can't move the sugar which is in your blood, into your cells. The blood sugar level rises.

Regular exercise stimulates and improves your cells ability to take in sugar, thus lowering your blood sugar level toward the normal range. Regular exercise such as walking or running will also help you to lose weight, decreasing the amount of insulin needed to keep your blood sugar in that normal range.

Overweight people are 250 percent more likely to develop diabetes. Most overweight, sedentary people have some degree of Insulin Resistance Syndrome, which is a precursor to diabetes.

Who else is affected by Type II Diabetes? Mostly the over 45s, overweight and inactive people. Type II diabetes runs in families too. Especially overweight, inactive families!

Lose enough weight and do enough exercise and you can control type II diabetes. According to a Finnish study, losing 10 pounds reduced the incidence of type II diabetes by 58 percent in those who were at high risk for diabetes. Prefer Harvard research?

30 minutes of exercise daily also reduced diabetes risk by 58 percent, reduced heart attack risk by 40 percent and female breast cancer risk by 30 percent. By the way, about 5 times more women die from diabetes related disease than from breast cancer.

Those nice Harvard people also say that a healthful breakfast such as whole-grain cereals, milk and fruit reduces diabetes risk by up to 50 percent.

Keep your BMI below 25, waistline under 35 inches and drink 4 to 5 cups of coffee to reduce your risk of diabetes. Eat 25 grams of fiber per day to further reduce your diabetes risk. Men should keep their waist measurement below 40 inches to reduce their diabetes and death risk.

BMI is your weight in kilograms divided by your height in meters...squared. Plug in pounds and inches at fitnessmagazine.com if you prefer.

Though high in calories and therefore the potential to give you weight gain, according to JAMA, Nov 27, 2,002, a tablespoon of peanut butter or ¼ cup of nuts on 5 days per week decreased diabetes risk by 20 to 30 percent. Replace croutons or other wasted carbs with the nuts of your choice and the protein and healthful fat will send the "don't need to eat for a while message" to your brain. Half the Americans who have diabetes don't know that they have it, so get yours checked.

6. Stronger bones & fewer fractures from osteoporosis.

According to the Journal of Bone and Mineral Research, vol. 12, 1997, women over the age of 50 who currently walk (or cycle out-doors) for more than 30 minutes a day are 20 % less likely to develop dowager's hump because of osteoporosis.

According to a study at Harvard Medical School by assistant professor Diane Feskanich, walk 4 or more hours per week and your hip fracture risk is 40 percent less than non-exercisers. Menopause puts women at risk for losing calcium and increases heart disease risk. Exercise reduces these menopausal risks.

Regain an additional one percent bone mass and you decrease your fracture risk by roughly 2 percent. Or, simply hold on to that one percent in the first place with exercise. Men who run 9 times per month have 8 percent greater bone density compared to inactive guys! Their fracture risk decreased by 16 percent.

Exercise involving gentle ground impact builds more bone than rhythmic exercise without ground impact. Running is better than cycling for preventing osteoporosis. Free weights are better than machines for building bone mass.

You'll need calcium too. The average person's consumption is 250 milligrams short of the RDA for calcium. Add an extra yogurt serving, or glass of non-fat milk to reach 1,200 mgs for the day. Munch on a tum if you need to save calories and avoid the other minerals and goodies from milk products.

Though vitamin K is better known for its blood clotting role, according to an analysis of my colleagues in the Nurses' Health Study, vitamin K is also important for bone health. You're 30 percent less likely to fracture a hip if you get your 109 micrograms of vitamin K per day. Collard greens, red cabbage, Brussel sprouts, spinach, broccoli, liver and eggs are good sources.

Most chocolate flavored calcium supplements include vitamin K, but get out and exercise too and your body will get the message to retain your calcium. You'll also need vitamin A made from your beta carotene and some vitamin D for healthy bones.

Regular exercise also decreases falls by 18 percent according to the Accident Research Center in Australia. Improve your strength and balance with exercise to decrease fractures.

7. Lower your Cholesterol.

According to a pilot study by Dr. Kraus at Duke University, exercising for one hour, four times per week for three months reduced low-density lipoprotein cholesterol (LDL) or bad cholesterol from 122 to 104 on average. High-density lipoprotein cholesterol (HDL) or good cholesterol rose from 32 to 37, making for huge gains in the HDL to LDL ratio from 3.81 to 2.81. You can also raise your HDL by 10 percent with three glasses of orange or cranberry juice per day. Any combination works, especially whole fruit. Half of adult Americans have high cholesterol.

The American Heart Association regards low levels of "good" cholesterol to be a risk factor for heart disease. HDL below 35 milligrams per deciliter increases your risk of a heart attack. You'll notice that the participants in the above study got their HDL up to

37. More than one in five men with heart disease suffer from low HDL despite having safe levels of LDL.

All people, especially people with low HDL should do aerobic exercise on a regular basis to raise their HDL levels. The result will be a reduction in the death rate from heart disease because HDL helps to clear out the arterial plaque which high LDL puts down.

Most of the statin drug family which lower cholesterol, can raise your blood sugar, making you more prone to diabetes. Statins are also apt to give you muscle weakness and rhabdomyolysis. Your MD needs to monitor your liver function with regular blood tests. Regular exercise makes your muscles stronger while taking your blood sugar closer to normal…and you need no blood tests!

Eating oatmeal, apples and whole-wheat products will also lower your cholesterol, while making your bowel movements more regular, which reduces your colon cancer risk. Aim for lots of water soluble fiber because it takes cholesterol out of your body; eat oats, beans, peas, barley, pears. Soy protein products like tofu and soy milk, also decrease cholesterol levels, as can fish oil. A little cinnamon can decrease your cholesterol and triglycerides, and also decrease your diabetes risk.

Eat a high fiber, near vegetarian diet to get huge decreases in your LDL level, which will also decrease your risk of osteopenia.

Almonds vitamin E, fiber and monounsaturated fat can reduce your LDL cholesterol by 7 percent, and keep you satiated for 90 minutes longer than non nut eaters. Up to two pints of beer per day can raise your HDL cholesterol by 12 percent. Both foods have lots of calories but can improve your LDL / HDL ratio. Oranges or OJ will also boost your HDLs.

Modest amounts of high calorie peanut butter can also improve your triglyceride levels, which further reduces your heart disease risk. Regular exercise will also reduce your triglyceride levels. Weight loss can give you a 10 percent drop in LDLs. Niacin can drop LDLs by 30 percent and raise your HDL by 20 percent. Use statins as the very last course.

Walnuts reduce your bloods stickyness by 20 percent, reducing the amount of plaque laid down in your arteries. 7 walnuts or one ounce contain enough omega-3 fatty acids for your hearts health.

8. Decrease belly fat and body weight.

According to the October 2,002 Journal of the American Medical Association, 64.5 percent of Americans are overweight. A 2001 Surgeon Generals report estimated that 300,000 deaths per year are due to obesity, especially items 1 and 2 of this appendix.

Regular running stimulates higher levels of fat-burning enzymes, increasing the amount of fat which you metabolize, especially during longer runs. So trim your belly with steady exercise. Build some muscle too because it will burn 40 to 50 calories per pound every day.

Regular exercise is vital to maintain ideal body weight. Fifteen to 30 percent of your energy expenditure each day is from physical activity. Achieve closer to 30 percent by running three miles per day and you'll expend an extra 300 plus calories and burn 30 pounds of fat per year.

According to a ten year study of 44,000 women, walking 4 or more hours a week reduced women's risk of gaining weight around their waists by 16%. Overweight men are 50 percent more likely to get heart disease than normal weight men.

Every year we hear of side effects from weight loss stimulants. The fen-phen debacle of the late 90s brought the problem a step further, the stimulant ephedra was banned by the FDA in April 2004, but quarana, ginseng, St. John's wort and melatonin are still available and causing side effects. Of course, despite its many uses, if aspirin sought FDA approval as a new drug in the last 10 years it probably would have been kept off the market.

The best way to lose belly fat is to exercise more and to eat less, using a low-fat diet. Make sure your low-fat substitutes are not high calorie due to massive amounts of sugar. Crunches and sit-ups will tone the muscles, but they burn very few calories. Any aerobic exercise for 40 minutes at modest intensity is the way to burn calories. Add minimal amounts of muscle with Chapter 16s weight training to burn even more calories every day.

Simple tricks can help you to lose weight. Starbucks serve up numerous 16 ounce mochas with whole milk and whipped cream at over 400 calories per serving! The 16 ounce non-fat cappuccino has a mere 110 calories. Have the mocha on Wednesdays because you still need a treat and some saturated fat, but save 290 calories on the other 4 work days per week to drop 17 pounds per year. The largest house coffee with 2 ounces of non-fat milk is a mere 23 calories! Check their nutritional handout to find other savings.

In a Harvard study of 74 thousand women, those who consumed more than two servings of whole grain were 49 percent less likely to be overweight than near fiber free white food eaters. Whole grains are absorbed slowly, giving less of an insulin reaction, take more calories to digest, and keep you feeling full longer.

Take in three serving of dairy and its calcium will make you 60 percent less likely to be overweight.

Healthful snacks made up of bulky carbohydrates like apples and bulky veggies such as broccoli, carrots and potatoes, also decrease the likelihood of you noshing on high calorie snacks like cookies. Although you'll want to include legumes such as peas for their protein and minerals, bulky vegetables are more filling and send the "I'm full signal" to your brain for fewer calories than legumes.

Start your exercise with water aerobics, weight training and biking to begin your weight loss. Fit but heavy people get the same health benefits as normal weight people. Get your body fat tested with calipers instead of only relying on weight or BMI. Once you've built some muscle, BMI is meaningless.

Dropping just 7 percent of their weight helped overweight people reduce signs of artery damage. You're more likely to lose weight with an exercise program if you also have nutritional advice and monitor and make small changes to your intake. Use Appendix II as a starting point.

9. Decrease eyesight loss from Glaucoma.

Exercise improves your eyesight. Glaucoma is the leading cause of vision loss and blindness in the U.S., and is the result of an increase in eye pressure. When sedentary people began a three times a week brisk walking program, those with glaucoma reduced their eye pressure by 20 percent. People without glaucoma also experienced a 9 percent reduction in eye pressure. (American Academy of Ophthalmology's annual meeting, Oct 1997).

10. Walking decreases the pain of arthritis.

Regular exercise stimulates thicker cartilage between your bones, and better muscle strength to keep your joints stable. Regular runners are five times less likely to have knee problems than sedentary folk and your spine and long bones will be 40 percent stronger. Running does not wear your body out. Runners have less disability than non-runners do. Your body is well designed for running, especially if you:

* Vary your pace from day to day;
* Run on different surfaces; and,
* Rotate three pairs of running shoes.

The musculoskeletal system adapts to increasing exercise levels but much slower than your cardiovascular system does. Train at 60 to 75 percent of your maximum heartrate to allow your muscles and bones to get stronger. Run at easy pace for several months, then begin graduated sessions of modest paced faster running.

Add strength training and balancing exercises to your running to decrease pain from arthritis and decrease risk of fractures.

And lose weight. Orthopedic nurses like myself have known for years that overweight people have more arthritis in weight bearing joints than normal weight people. Now the scientists tell us it is partly due to leptin, which is released from fat cells. And it affects non weight bearing joints too. According to Boston University, every additional kilogram (2.2 pounds) lost decreases osteoarthritis risk by 9 to 13 percent, and by 50 percent for a 5 kg or 11 pound loss. Weight loss also decreases your leptin levels, which decreases risk of arthritis and joint deformity. Of course, weight loss will also decrease arthritis symptoms if you already have the disease.

Weight loss also decreases your rheumatoid arthritis symptoms, but exercise mostly with pool running, biking, and elliptical training, plus stretching and weight training to make the best of your immune systems cruelty.

Include some omega-3s from cold water fish or fish oil capsules or flaxseed oil to further reduce inflammatory diseases like rheumatoid arthritis and arterial diseases. Reduce decaf coffee consumption if your concern is rheumatoid arthritis. Pineapple juice also helps many people via its anti-inflammatory, bromelain. Chondroitin sulfate supplements helps many people with sore joints, including the back, by rebuilding your cartilage.

Fibromyalgia responds in a nasty way to over exercise, but responds well to gentle exercise at the right level for your muscles (some people call fibromyalgia arthritis of the muscles). Check to see if you have enough vitamin D in your system and then experiment to find out the right types of exercise for you.

11. Run to increase your libido.

Able to exercise for an hour at a time, with good circulation to your heart and other muscles? You'll have good circulation to your sex glands too. Vigorous exercise increases hormone levels and boosts self-confidence in men and women. Men's testosterone levels rise after a 30 minute run and stay up for 60 minutes! Plan on running with your partner, even if one of you rides a bike while the other runs. Weight training also raises testosterone levels, which will make you less likely to have a stroke.

You're 30 percent less likely to have erectile dysfunction if you do the equivalent of 18 miles of running per week. Lean men and men with low amounts of TV watching also have fewer problems.

Remember to consume sufficient zinc to assist your activity. Because you sweat out a bit of zinc, you'll need about 15 mg per day to keep your testosterone and sperm counts up, plus for your red blood cells and for bone strength. A pair of oysters would supply your daily need, but most breakfast cereals are fortified with 25 percent of your zinc needs per serving and you'll also get substantial zinc from meats (6 mg per 3 ounces of steak), your milk products (3 mg per serving), Lentils at 2 mg per half cup, whole grain products and cashew nuts.

Aiming for conception? Consume 500 milligrams of vitamin C spread though out the day, including several servings of fruit, to decrease the percentage of sperm which stick together. Men who consume 500 mgs of vitamin C also live longer. If you're overweight, you'll have more damaged sperm.

There is a direct correlation between hypertension in the form of high blood pressure and hypertension in the form of stress, so get control of these two. Erectile dysfunction is a subtle warning sign for heart disease.

12. Exercise elevates your mood.

Regular exercise is an effective way to release tension and reduce anxiety. Exercise increases the level of the neurotransmitter serotonin in your brain, which elevates your mood. Exercise also uses up some of those debilitative fight or flight chemicals. Exercise reduces your stress levels, releases muscle tension and has fewer side effects than sedatives! Longer runs allow you to release even more stress, but build up to them gradually.

Beat depression: According to research at Duke University, 30 minutes of moderate running three days a week is as effective as medication for the clinically depressed. Exercisers also improved concentration, planning and organization. There are unpleasant side effects from prozac and other pills. The main side effect from exercise is a stronger heart to cope with life's problems.

Getting started? Ten minutes of exercise will improve your mood according to a study in the July 2001 issue of Health Psychology. Not used to exercise? Keep the exercise intensity and duration low for the first few sessions. Gradually increase the duration and then the intensity as your fitness and mood improves.

Clear your mind and get an attitude adjustment on a daily basis, but not with running every day: take a bike ride or a walk on the beach or in a park. Exercising in sunlight releases even more beta-endorphins to make you feel good. Avoid the gym when you can.

Runners know that the glass of life is at least half full and rarely see it as half empty. They have a positive outlook on life partly because running is a positive achievement.

Many of the 18 million depressed Americans use depression as an excuse for overeating to console themselves. These comfort foods then make them more depressed due to reduction in self-esteem. Eat your veggies for the folate and cold water fish too. Don't overdo your consumption of predatory large fish like tuna shark and swordfish or your brain may go fussy from mercury.

Had a tough day sitting at your desk? You will feel more energetic after a run than before it. Run at the right pace for you and for the right amount of time based on recent runs to relieve the stress from your day or your life. Been physically active at work? You still need 30 minutes of aerobic activity for your heart and brain. For each hour per week of exercise, you'll reduce your risk of depression by 8 percent.

13. Increased cognitive function.

If you've been inactive for 40 plus years, you can still regain mental acuity. Studies at University of Illinois with formerly sedentary 60-75 year olds showed improvement in concentration, planning, and organization. Late life exercising is better than no exercising. It is never too late to start exercising.

After the age of 30, our brain tissue begins to deteriorate. Over the next 60 years roughly 25 percent of the memory, learning and thinking parts of the brain are lost. According to researchers at the University of Illinois, MRIs of cardiovascularly fit people had more gray and white matter than non-exercisers. What does it matter that fit people have more matter left? The white matter transmits signals; the gray matter is vital for learning and memory.

It doesn't matter if you declined to enter 5K races or neglected to reach 40 minute runs. What matters is that you exercise for 20 minutes on three to four days each week. Most of the other health benefits are not reached until you're doing a total of 3 to 4 hours per week of exercise though, and you're likely to be even more alert (i.e. alive) at age 90 if you average 40 minutes per day of exercise. Regular exercise also makes you 33 percent less likely to get Alzheimer's disease.

Most of this book is based on a goal of 40 minutes exercise on 5 days per week but the 2,003 guidelines for humans is 60 minutes of exercise every day. Only 13 % of women reach 30 minutes per day and only 15 % of men get 30 minutes, so while exercise is good for your body and your head, you have to set the limit.

14. Less breast cancer.

Regular exercise decreases breast cancer risk by at least 20 percent. According to the Archives of Internal Medicine, nurses who exercised more than 7 hours per week had 20 percent less breast cancer than nurses who did less than one hour of vigorous exercise. Sustained walking is sufficient. Walking to your patient and giving patient care is a more active pastime than working at a desk! Walking to your colleague instead of sending an e-mail is fitness enhancing and more sociable.

Exercise can alleviate the pain which some people with cancer get, and give you a positive achievement every time you exercise.

Exercise at moderate intensity also decreases the fatigue from cancer therapy: you're better prepared to tolerate your treatments. Exercise even decreases lymphedema, the pesky inflammation which sometimes occurs after surgery.

According to the Journal of the National Cancer Institute, Nov 20, 2002, obese women secrete more leptin, a hormone which makes cancer cells grow 3 times faster. Exercise to maintain a healthy weight (waist below 28 inches) to reduce your leptin production. If you're overweight, lose 20 pounds to decrease breast cancer risk by 21 percent.

The above holds true for most cancers. You're less likely to get ovarian cancer if you consume low amounts of simple or refined sugars. Complex carbohydrate from whole veggies and fruit with its cancer-fighting beta carotene can give you a cancer fighting edge, as does consuming fish, flaxseed oil or ground flaxseed and soy products. Calcium and vitamin D decreases colon cancer risk. Daily citrus intake cuts your risk of oral and stomach cancer.

Seven aspirin tabs per week can also reduce breast cancer risk by 28 percent. Aspirin decreases estrogen levels, decreases colon cancer, but its main longevity benefit is from decreased circulation disease due to its effect on platelets and as an anti inflammatory on blood vessels.

An hour per day of exercise such as walking also lowers your risk of endometrial cancer by 30 percent.

15. Exercise reduces Tylenol needs.

Aerobic exercise reduces chronic headaches by reducing stress, increasing your endorphins, (a natural analgesic), and by decreasing insomnia. Regular exercisers decrease their Tylenol needs.

Overdosing on acetaminophen, which is the active ingredient in Tylenol was responsible for 39 percent of acute liver failure cases in a 2,002 study. Most overdoses were accidental. Acetaminophen is in cough and cold medicines, is used to aid sleep and for pain. It's easy to amass 4,000 milligrams a day of this liver destroyer, though small people will have their liver damaged at lower doses.

16. Save your stomach too.

Non Steroidal Anti-Inflammatory Drugs (NSAIDs) such as aspirin and ibuprofen crop up in numerous cold remedies too. Wonderful for short-term use for pain and to reduce muscle and joint inflammation, continued use will decrease the lining of the stomach and increase the risk of ulcers.

Over 16 thousand deaths per year are linked to NSAID use, so don't take them for a chronic problem. Find the cause of your chronic pains and back off from training. Don't take pain pills before exercise and don't take them on an empty stomach.

The fairly new cox-2 inhibitors have been touted as gentler to the stomach. However, researchers in the December 26th 2,002 issue of the New England Journal reported that nearly 10 percent of users who were at risk for ulcers developed bleeding ulcers while taking celebrex. Vioxx and Bextra are likely to give the same results. These drugs also increase the risk of renal insufficiency.

17. Problems with Insomnia...exercise is better than a Restoril or other sedative.

Regular aerobic exercise such as walking or running improves the quality of your sleep and decreases the time that it takes to fall asleep. Improving the quality of content or the duration makes you more alert and happier. Improving both can make you more productive at work and content during your active hours. Exercise for 40 minutes at modest intensity, 2 to 4 hours before you wish to sleep. Include Turkey or milk in your snack for their tryptophan.

18. Exercise for your baby.

Do moderately intensive weight bearing exercise on several days per week during early pregnancy and you'll improve fetoplacental growth rates. Your baby and you will be healthier during and after the birth. You'll be fitter to cope with the birthing process and your recovery will be faster. You're more likely to need a C-section if you are overweight, or if you gain more than 40 pounds during pregnancy. Maintain a gentle exercise schedule for your entire pregnancy to keep both of you healthy. The overweight are also less likely to conceive and more likely to have a miscarriage.

After the birth, you may want to stay mainly with cross training. The hormone relaxin increases elasticity in joints and ligaments, which is very nice during childbirth, but can make it easier to strain joints and muscles afterwards. For a few weeks you'll still be carrying a bit of extra weight, so give your joints a chance by biking, elliptical training and pool running before venturing back to the running trails.

19. Exercise reduces Deep Vein Thrombosis (DVTs).

DVTs kill 60,000 Americans every year. Inactivity such as office work and sitting on an airplane increases your risk of DVTs. Actually, the DVT is merely the precursor to your death. A piece of that clot which breaks off and whips through your heart to your lungs is your death plug or nail. The clot settles in a pulmonary artery to become a pulmonary embolism (PE). Shortness of breath, sudden chest pain, dizziness and fainting make it hard to distinguish a PE from a myocardial infarction. No worries though because you'll be rushed to hospital anyway, and several of the treatments such as clot busting drugs are the same.

When blood volume has been stabilized after an operation, early ambulation and gentle range of motion exercises are the keys to preventing blood clots in the large leg muscles, and also decreases the risk of pneumonia. The walking also enhances mood and recovery from the surgery.

Don't wait for a major operation to get your legs moving. Walk a few hundred yards several times a day, especially when on long journeys. Get a 40 minute moderately intensive exercise session most days. Walk a few hundred feet at the end of runs and stay hydrated to decrease your DVT and PE risk. Drinking 16 ounces of water can also raise your metabolism by 30 percent for over an hour, so helping your weight control (saves soda calories too).

20. Use exercise to beat smoking.

Walk one block every time you feel like smoking and take nicotine from medicinal sources (patch, gum or chewing tobacco) to break the initial habit. When you've overcome the psychological need for nicotine, such as the burning feeling you get when you destroy another chunk of your lung with your most recent inhalation, ease off on the medicinals to decrease your physiological nicotine needs. Exercise 5 days per week for up to 40 minutes to clear your lungs.

21. Exercise to Grow Younger.

70-year-olds who weight train and do aerobic exercise have the muscle strength and endurance of average 30 year olds.

30-year-olds lose about 12 percent of their maximum oxygen uptake or aerobic ability every decade. Runners lose less than half of their oxygen use ability. Inactivity leads to half of your physiological aging. The passage of time does lead to chronological ageing, but does relatively little to age you physiologically if you remain active.

Include weight training just twice each week to maintain most of your muscle mass, while keeping your metabolism up and preventing the addition of unwanted fatty tissue.

22. Exercise away your asthma.

Start at extremely low intensity with a prolonged warm up to prevent an asthma attack during exercise. Then incorporate 3 to 4 minute efforts at 30 to 40 seconds slower than 5K pace to fully open your airways. Warmdown fully and remember to carry your emergency puffer for the occasional day when you do things too quickly. Warm air and early morning is the best combination for your exercise session.

23. Don't overheat and epileptics can exercise.

Improve your health with exercise and you may decrease your risk of seizures. But don't overheat or dehydrate.

24. Exercise to decrease PMS.

Physical symptoms of Premenstrual Syndrome include headache, fluid retention, fatigue, painful joints and backache, abdominal cramping, weight gain and heart palpitations. Mood swings, anxiety, panic attacks, tension and depression may also be present. As you've read above, moderate intensity exercise, including running can decrease almost all of those symptoms.

Studies show that daily 1,200 mgs of calcium or 30 minutes of exercise can reduce PMS symptoms. Oddly enough, the RDA for calcium is 1,200 mgs, which is increased to 1,500 when you're pregnant or when you've surpassed the chronological age of 51.

25. Exercise to force away the winter blues.

Seasonal Affective Disorder (SAD) is a form of depression due to a lack of sunlight, usually in winter and in the northern states. SAD is also used as an excuse to overindulge in carbohydrates, yet if you get outside for half an hour most lunchtimes and if football or basketball are your passions, watch it outside or play them yourself, you should decrease your risk of feeling SAD. Get outside soon after you wake up.

To paraphrase a recent article on the subject, SAD makes you feel sad. SAD also lowers your sex drive, makes you less affective at work and makes you sleepy. As you know from 11 & 17 above, regular exercise reverses those problems.

Wear a teashirt most days and sunscreen on exposed parts and your skin cancer risk is not increased…provided you also avoid sunburn. A sunlamp will not cause sunburn either, because it filters out UV rays. Waiting around on race day for the results? Wear a hat and refresh your sunscreen.

26. Cope with Irritable Bowel System (IBS).

Studies show that physically active people have a better quality of life and cope better with their IBS. According to a University of Pittsburgh study, IBS sufferers should consume 25 or more grams of fiber, plus plenty of water. Still no relief after a couple of months? Consider Paxil to cut some of the intestinal spasms.

Regular exercise also decreases your risk of diverticular disease and helps you to cope with many other diseases including multiple sclerosis.

27. Run to beat that Cold.

Regular exercise decreases your common cold risk because you're healthier. Exercise makes it easier for you to recover from a cold because your immune cells circulate at a higher rate. You can also go running with a cold, but a severe bout of the flu, weakness or a chest infection generally require a rest from running. Don't increase your exercise while you have a cold or illness. Stay hydrated and do a bit less than usual and at a lower intensity. As mentioned earlier, exercise stimulates the production of Human Growth Hormone, which ultimately helps you to fight colds and other infections.

The secrets to gaining health benefits from exercise are not remotely secret:

* Exercise regularly based on a specific plan;
* Exercise at a moderate intensity for the middle section;
* Exercise for 40 minutes or more, five or six days a week;
* Picture yourself getting fitter and healthier.
* While enjoying 95 % of the exercise you do (sometimes, a few minutes will need to seem a little tough).
* Do a variety of exercises from chapters 16 & 17 plus running.

Remember to start your exercise program gently because your muscles and bones adapt to exercise slower than your heart and lungs do. Look again at the cartoon on page 28. Don't hurt yourself people, because you'll be exercising again tomorrow.

The next section is on nutrition, but first a few benefits of consuming caffeine and coffee.

<u>Coffee</u> consumption, provided it's in a low calorie format, decreases your risk of being overweight and it's slew of related diseases like cardiac arrest. Note: officially it's heart <u>disease</u> and one of the symptoms is cardiac arrest. Coffee also decreases your gallstone risk, diabetes and Parkinson's disease. Decaf does not help, but the caffeine in tea helps decrease risk of some diseases.

If these caffeinated drinks keep you away from the fructose in sodas and fruit cocktails you'll weigh less. If they are taken in conjunction with milk, they'll produce a smaller blood sugar spike, while also giving you numerous antioxidants.

About 4 servings of coffee give you the maximum benefits, but you should also get your 40 minutes of exercise 5 days per week and monitor calorie intake to be your ideal weight.

Caffeine is not dehydrating unless you're only consuming triple shots in 4 ounce cups and no other liquids.

Appendix II

A bit(e) on Nutrition

Although this authors e-book *301 Balanced Eating & Nutrition Tips* is a fine resource for advice, I owe it to you to give a few key eating tips. As that book says, nutrition, not dieting is the best approach to avoid weight gain or achieve weight loss. Most people who successfully keep weight off are a little bit careful about what they eat and exercise regularly.

Changing your behavior is one key to weight loss. Two 22 ounce beers and a hamburger and fries, plus bar snacks, clearly contain more calories than one 12 ounce beer and a *Healthy Choice* Salisbury steak meal, plus half a cantaloupe. Neither options require that you cook. The second option keeps you reasonably sober and saves you over 40 minutes to exercise. Hint: Exercise, drink some water and then eat the meal.

Other behavior calorie savers include:

o   Staying away from snack machines;
o   Spending less time with overweight friends, or meeting them in a park for a slow walk.
o   Monitoring what goes into your belly: plain popcorn is better than potato chips. Don't double the financial cost of a movie with popcorn and soda.
o   Write down what you eat in a food diary for several days to find your habits. Locate the wasted fat and the other calories which give you negligible pleasure.
o   Keep unhealthful food choices out of your house.
o   Figure out the stimuli which make you eat and find a past-time or hobby to do during potential binging time. No emotional eating; it solves nothing.

If you watch commercial television, you've seen Jared and friends with their "subway" weight loss. At a mere 300 calories or under,

Subway has seven sandwiches with protein and veggies to see you through the next 4 hours, or add an hour by eating a piece of fruit with your 6-inch sub. Tempted by the meatball sandwich? You'll clock up 527 calories. Forget the Atkins or low carb wrap, it packs 480 calories and 27 grams of fat.

Avoid the mayo and other dressings, and most fast food places can match subway. For instance, Burger King's veggie burger has 330 calories; its Chicken Whopper Junior (yes runners, adults are allowed to eat them) is 350 calories and its Junior hamburger w/o mayo is 310 calories. The drawback is the availability of French fries at 300 plus calories in most places and soft drinks at 200 calories per medium cup.

At home, the actual veggie burger has ample protein, usually soy which is good for you, and saves 120 calories compared to beef. Lean Cuisine, Healthy Choice, Weight Watchers and others such as Uncle Bens produce 300 to 400 calorie meals in reasonably low fat options. Add a serving of fruit and a couple of small potatoes without fat on them or whole wheat bread to make them balanced meals.

If you don't allow yourself to get really hungry, you're less likely to pig out. Go food shopping just after dinner and you'll avoid the crowds and be less likely to pick up sweet foods.

* Eat a calcium and protein containing breakfast plus some carbs, and you're one-quarter of the way to healthful eating techniques. (Your body gets the message that you have taken in two vital nutrients and you get fewer messages to eat later in the day. You burn more calories, yet make fewer fat cells.)

* Keep healthful snacks such as fruit and low fat energy bars on hand at work and keep lots of whole-grain foods at home and you're half-way there.

* Don't buy ice-cream and other high fat foods like chips and T-bone steaks (instead, eat 3 ounce portions of lean meats like eye-of-round beef, white chicken or turkey meat without the skin, or fish) and you're three-quarters of the way there.

* Sound hydration and eating plenty of fruit and vegetables gives you your remaining quarter.

You can still eat an occasional treat, but don't have them so handily available that they become a staple of your food intake.

Calories are the key to weight control. Nutritionists
agree: Take in too many calories per year and you'll gain weight. Eat a small amount of quality protein and some bulky carbohydrates 4 to 5 times per day while moderating the high fat types of protein such as peanut butter, oils and spreads and you've got a good chance of controlling your weight. Ignore the net carbs fad (the FDA has). Read how many calories your food contains.

The energy needed to metabolize food and drink or the "thermic effect of food," burns 10 percent of your calories. Eat many small meals, eat breakfast, include fiber and you'll burn more calories.

Broccoli, cabbage, green beans, carrots, tomatoes and actual apples contain many nutrients but fewer calories than peas, beans, corn and apple juice. While you can also consume the last four options, most of the first group are likely to take you longer to eat and give you a feeling of fullness earlier than the second group. The fiber or roughage as we called it in the 1970s, will keep your intestines in good order. Cruciferous veggies like broccoli and cabbage also reduce your risk of bladder cancer by 50 percent.

Don't go overboard about avoiding high glycemic index foods. Sure, the sugar in a bag of carrots gets into the bloodstream pretty fast, but you're unlikely to eat more than three ounces of them, which is a nutritious 38 calorie bargain.

A three ounce piece of low fat meat or glass of non-fat milk or yogurt will complement the fruits and veggies, but you'll still need some wholesome energy source for your complex carbs.

Potatoes, whole-wheat breads or whole-wheat pasta and raw foods are better for you than processed or manufactured white foodstuffs such as white rice and white bread. Duran wheat is used for most types of pasta and provided you eat large types, the glycemic index is below 50.

Ready for dessert? Dip into the calcium group for non-fat yogurt. Studies show that people who consume adequate amounts of calcium are less likely to over consume calories. Calcium consumers also burn more fat and store less fat. But watch out. A low fat yogurt has 250 calories. A lite yogurt has only 100 calories. Eat a medium size banana instead of chips for a huge saving.

One glass of tomato juice will supply more electrolytes than four glasses of Gatorade for only 25 percent of the calories. The tomato juice also has vitamins, a spot of protein and fiber and goes well with a wheat bagel and water for a balanced snack after a 60 minute run. Only need the electrolytes? You've just saved 150 calories by drinking tomato juice; drink some water to complete your hydration. Save those 150 calories after 5 runs per week and you'll lose 11 pounds this year, and 11 pounds next year. The lycopene in tomato products also protects against cancers.

Fruit juices contains huge amounts of calories. Use a tall, thin glass and you'll poor less juice. Avoid fruit blends saturated with fructose. Whole fruits such as the melon family including cantaloupe, plus oranges, berries and grapes provide substantial amounts of liquid while also supplying antioxidants to fight the free radicals in your system. A cup of fruit has fewer calories than a cup of fruit juice.

64.5 percent of U.S. adults are overweight.

Too much fat on your body will slow down your running. Take control of your eating. It's you who is putting it into your mouth, so stop those excuses.

It's OK to run while your overweight because you get the same health benefits as normal weight people, yet by decreasing your intake by 250 calories a day, you will lose a pound every two weeks. Avoid or decrease the following mistakes:

* Don't rush. Smell, chew and savor your meals.
* Second helpings, especially of desserts save 250 calories;
* Second and subsequent beers or wine at 100 to 200 calories.
* Low carb or lite (or light) beer? There is hardly any calorie difference, as most of the calories come from the alcohol. Drink one can or bottle of the type which satisfies you.
* Regular soda at over 100 to 140 calories for every 12 ounces; 250 calories for a bottle of regular coke. Switch to diet soda.
* Hold the cheese on hamburgers;
* Hold the mayo on hamburgers to save 90 calories (at home you can use fat-free mayo, but check the calorie count!)
* Avoid those big muffins to save 200 to 300 calories;
* Fatty or high calorie salad dressing; olive oil and nut based oils are unsaturated and contain no trans-fatty acids: keep it at the side of your salad instead of dripping it over the salad.

* Regular or decaf coffee with a little non-fat milk will save 200 calories compared to a bottle of refrigerated coffee.
* Eat a cereal bar instead of a bagel with cream cheese on some days to save over 160 calories.
* Low sugar does not mean low calorie. Check the label.
* Eat your 3 ounces of shrimp in a shrimp cocktail instead of breaded and fried to save 120 calories.
* Butter-flavored flakes instead of butter saves 100 calories.
* Grill off the fat from your lean meat instead of frying it in fat to save 200 calories per portion. Pop your own corn to control the portion, and use no butter to save hundreds of calories.
* Fudge covered cookies cost about 225 calories per pair. Cut an energy bar in half, zip-lock one half and save 70-100 calories.
* Recipes: Cut 30 % of the sugar; use half the recommended fat but substitute canola or olive oil for butter or margarine; use predominantly egg whites instead of whole eggs; it's possible to make healthful foods tasty.
* Real raspberries or strawberries have fewer calories than their sorbets, though sorbet often has fewer calories than ice cream. The July 2,004 *Prevention* magazine tested what they titled "Healthy Frozen Treats" The low carb Vanilla ice cream had more calories than 5 of the other suggestions, but 9 grams of fat. Smart Ones Fudge bars have 50 percent fewer calories (80), zero fat and a respectable 4 grams of fiber.
* Turkey hot dogs have 135 fewer calories than beef dogs.
* Roast chicken has 75 less calories per portion than fried.
* Use low fat cheese.
* Some days you'll want corn and beans for carbs, protein and calories. Other days look to carrots, broccoli and other bulky veggies to fill you up at low calorie cost.

Change some of the above each day for significant calorie savings. The exercise you are doing each day will help you to maintain muscle and help you to lose weight.

Looking for Quicker Weight Loss

Lose five pounds in 5 days on the THREE shakes a day Hollywood style diets…provided you burn 4,250 calories per day. Alas, most people who need to lose weight burn less than 2,000 per day, which is half of the reason they are overweight. The second half is over-consumption of food.

To lose a pound of fat you need to burn 3,500 calories. Add in the 750 calories from those three shakes, and you have to burn 4,250 calories to one pound per day. Yet advertisers still make their weight loss claim. The actual (short-term) weight lose is mostly from the shunting of fluid which occurs when you suddenly deny yourself food. Starving yourself will use up some of your glycogen stores, which contains prodigious amounts of water.

The day you re-commence normal eating, the glycogen stores, and the water, is restored. Follow the advice in *5K Fitness Walk*: make subtle changes to your eating habits.

Protein Debate:

Building muscle requires protein but not supplements. Most people in western society get more than 150 percent of the recommended daily allowance (RDA) for protein. Eat a balanced diet with a quality protein source 4 to 5 times per day and you'll have plenty of the building bricks (amino acids) to form large muscles. You'll gain less than an ounce (28 grams) per day of muscle with weight training. Hardly any of those 28 grams are protein, so 75 to 105 grams of protein daily will give you plenty of bricks. A high protein diet is dehydrating and it's cruel to your kidneys and your heart. The *late* Atkins diet should join him in the grave. It gets only 5 percent of its calories from carbohydrate, which is insufficient to power your brain, let alone your other muscles!

28 grams of most meats supply 7 grams of protein, as does an egg white, half a cup of cooked beans, ¾ cup of yogurt or skimmed milk, 2/3 rds of a whole wheat bagel or 1.5 cups of wheat chex.

Consume the mortar too: Fruit and vegetables keep you healthy. Fill up with these goodies for tons of Vitamins, minerals and antioxidants and phytochemicals. Citrus fruits, berries, kiwi and the melon clan, green and yellow veggies, beans and grains give a foundation to your carbohydrate and vitamin intake.

Carbohydrate is vital for running because its sugar is converted to glycogen and ATP (Adenosine Triphosphate). ATP is the energy source which muscles use to power their contractions, but even in well trained muscles, ATP is in short supply. Sugar in the bloodstream and glycogen in the muscles and liver are required to constantly replenish the ATP as it is used during running. Feed yourself with 60 percent of calories from complex carbohydrates and you'll get plenty of fuel to your muscle fibers.

Take in more than the recommended 5 fruits and veggies to get your carbs in a healthful way.

One kilocalorie will allow your muscles to produce sufficient ATP to propel you about 15 yards. 120 calories will get most people a mile of locomotion. Unless you're running for over an hour, you should not need to ingest carbos during exercise.

Take in up to 20 percent of your calories as protein and the remainder by default will be fat. On 2,000 calories per day you have 44 grams of fat to play with: make sure it's mostly from veggies to avoid the cholesterol, from fish with its omega-3 fatty acids for your heart and from monounsaturated sources like olive oil or canola oil. Consider Enova oil too. Decrease saturated fat intake (meat and regular milk products) and avoid trans fat (in solid oils like margarine and processed foods such as cookies).

Iron is essential for oxygen transport, so you might want to get your blood iron, serum ferritin, and hemoglobin levels checked on a yearly basis. Anemia also decreases your healing and recovery capacity, making you more prone to injury. Iron is poorly absorbed in the presence of caffeine, so split your iron source and caffeine drinks by 2 hours. Consume a vitamin C source at the same time as your iron packed food (lean red meats, dark poultry meat, beans and other legumes) to triple the percentage of iron absorbed. The iron in soy beans and its products is in the form of ferritin, which the body absorbs easier than other plant sources of iron. Make sure you get sufficient Folic acid and B12. (Insufficient B12 also raises homocysteine levels, a risk factor for heart disease.)

Recovery Snacks.

Drinking non-fat milk, yogurt smoothies or eating low fat energy bars straight after exercise helps muscles to recover from all types of training. Your muscles respond well to a quick hit of carbos and a little protein to begin their recovery. Gentle aerobic exercise after weight sessions also flushes your muscles with nutrient rich blood and sets you up for your next workout in which you give a moderate stress to a different aspect of your fitness.

Use any style of non-fat milk, including chocolate, or yogurt, or non-fat soy milk or tofu for your smoothie's protein source. Three servings of whole fruit and some ice chips, then blend, and you've got 75 grams or so of carbohydrate, plus 10 to 15 grams of protein to start your muscles re-fueling. Texture the smoothie to your taste.

Eight ounces of frozen strawberries for only 75 calories is a convenient way to make the smoothie cold. Eight large, fresh ones are 50 calories. Milk or yogurt plus a banana gives texture, protein and more carbos, then add almost any other ingredient for variety. Add a few ounces of tofu or more fat-free yogurt to make your smoothie into a protein snack if it is a meal replacement, and get a ton of B vitamins by adding a tablespoon of wheat germ.

A cup of non-fat milk is also useful just before weight training to give you some sugar for lifting and amino acids to improve your protein synthesis. A balanced snack close to bed-time will also keep your muscles happy, as will a sensible low fat breakfast.

Too busy for breakfast? Quaker 1-minute oats or sachets of oatmeal are almost as fast as wheat chex or other high fiber cereals, or get up two minutes earlier and do whole wheat toast.

Hint: Whole wheat or whole grain should be the first ingredient listed for your bread, and it should contain at least 2 grams of fiber per slice or serving. Whole grain breads and products contain about 20 more nutrients than white bread, including its germ, bran, B vitamins, vitamin E, zinc, magnesium, chromium, selenium and anti-cancer and heart healthy phytochemicals and antioxidants.

Set the alarm two minutes earlier to peel an orange for its fiber instead of drinking OJ. Many breakfast bars are packed with calcium, soy protein and fiber. Or drink an instant breakfast shake with its pureed fruit and soy protein, followed by an apple.

Unless you're fasting for the rest of the day, you don't need 100 percent of your RDA for any nutrient at breakfast, though it's prudent to consume 50 percent of your calcium needs (see below). Find your trigger points for overeating, then make pre-emptive strikes by eating a healthful snack half an hour before that time. If you're overweight, never eat in front of the TV.

Avoid fad diets which make you cut out an entire food group, or which limit you to say three specific foods for 7 days. Both systems do restrict your calories, but make eating boring due to lack of choice. Denial just leads to rebound eating later.

Taking in zero food after 7 pm is cute, and stops you eating in front of the TV and other snacky opportunities, but starving your muscles for 12 hours is not prudent. However, as will take about 4 hours for your dinner to be fully absorbed, if you finish dinner at 7 pm, and run at 6 am, you've only gone 7 hours without feeding your muscle fibers.

Take a 150 calorie snack such as non-fat yogurt or 12 ounces of 1 % milk before bed will mean a mere 3 to 4 hours that your physiological system does not have food coming in to prepare for exercise and to decrease hunger pangs in the morning. Have a glass of non-fat milk before your early run and your muscles and liver will laugh with their over supply of energy. These snacks also supply protein and calcium for muscle and bone building.

A low carb diet is simply another name for a high protein and or high fat diet. The zone and other low carb diets deny your muscles the energy to shift your body across the planet. Fat and protein are poor energy sources.

Take in complex carbs such as whole wheat bread, beans and potatoes, bear in mind that net carbs or impact carbs are just gimmicks and that low carb foods often have more calories than regular foods and you'll do fine in the ads versus reality stakes. Example: Regular ice cream is full of fat and has modest amounts of carbohydrate. Low carb ice cream has even more fat. One measuring cup of cooked pasta and rice have 200 and 170 calories respectively. You have to control how many cups you eat and how much fat you put on top to avoid weight gain.

If you drink two regular sodas every day, changing to one diet soda and one glass of non-fat milk will save over 150 calories per day, or 16 pounds per year.

The protein and calcium in the milk will also decrease the likelihood of you overeating later. Calcium intake has a direct correlation to body weight according to many studies released in 2,002 and 2,003. Consuming calcium causes the body to make less fat, yet it increases the bodies ability to break down fat. Choose low fat sources for calcium and see Osteoporosis in Appendix I.

I said it was a quick look at food. Want full calorie and nutrient info? Try www.nal.usda.gov/fnic/cgi-bin/nut_search.pl
Or check this author's 5K Walking or the DASH diet at:
www.nhlbi.nih.gov/health/public/heart/hbp/dash

Long Term Weight Loss is rarely successful with dietary changes alone. You will need to exercise to help lose weight and to keep it off.

Swimming burns about 100 calories for every 500 yards, or 20 lengths of a 25 yard pool. Switch to pool running after your swim to burn more calories with your leg muscles.

Walking burns a very nice 100 calories per mile…even more if you're overweight or walk in sand, or up hill or fast (because you're less efficient). Of course, that mile in sand or up hill will take you longer to walk. Running takes less time per mile.

Weigh in at 140 pounds? Here's your approximate calorie burn when exercising at moderate intensity.

Walk or run   100 calories per mile;
Swim   500 yards for 100 calories;
Biking   15 minutes for 100 calories;
Stair Climber   15 minutes per 100 calories;
Elliptical Trainer   15 minutes per 100 calories;
Rowing or cross country ski machine   11 minutes for 100 calories;
Elliptical machine with arm movement   11 mins = 100 calories
Weight training   204 calories for 30 minutes
Walking could also be 43 calories per 10 minutes;
Jumping rope or other plyometrics - 100 calories per 10 minutes;
Stretching is a modest 45 per 15 minute session.

Do those exercises efficiently and you'll burn fewer calories, but with less injury risk. Don't expect the exercise machine at the gym to accurately tell you how many calories you burn. Like the numbers above, they will only get to within 20 % of your calorie burn. Combine exercise with calorie control for steady weight loss.

Check www.shape.com/tools   for an additional number for your everyday and exercise activities.

Appendix III

Staying in your Heartrate Training Zone.

Adapted from pages 91-92 and 105-107 of Best Half-Marathons. Long repeats keep you in your training zone for a greater percentage of your training time.

When running 400 meter repeats, a person with a maximum exercise HR of 175 may only reach his 5K HR of 166 for the last 40 to 50 meters of each Interval. Here's the HR splits for 100s during a 400 meters. 148, 159, 164, 167.

This athlete was running slightly faster than 5K pace, so gaining very good skills at economical running, yet his heart was only at 5K intensity for about 10 percent of his Interval training. What happens if our hero slows down to 5K pace, but runs 800s?

Distance	HR	HR
200	159	157
400	164	163
600	169	169
800	171	167
Finish time	2.50	2.53

That 167 HR at the end of the second repeat was a reflection of our runner slowing down. Observe:

* Slightly lower HR at 400 meters secondary to slower running (compared to his earlier 400s).
* But he was only seconds away from hitting his 5K HR goal of 166 at the end of the first lap, and spent over 300 meters above 166 (40 percent of his Interval training).
* If he took shorter recoveries, he could reach his 166 HR goal earlier in each repeat, though this would make the session feel and be harder. Your goal should be to gradually reduce your rest periods.

Moving up to 1,600 meter repeats, lets see how much time you can spend in the training zone while at 5K pace, using a 400 meter rest in three minutes for the recovery.

	Heartrate for		
At	1st rep	2nd	3rd
200 m	154	154	159
400	162	164	162
600	163	166	164
800	164	169	165
1,200	166	169	167
1,600	169	168	166

He reaches his 10K HR goal of 161 well before the 400 meter point. If you run mile repeats at 5K pace, you'll probably get over 80 % of your Interval time at or above 10K heartrate intensity, or 92 % of max HR. 400s at 5K pace give you less than 30 percent of your time at 10K HR or higher.

But the main interest here is on 5K heartrate. During the first rep in this session, he took nearly 1,200 meters to reach his 5K heartrate (166 or more) with fresh legs. However, after a three minute rest, he took less than 600 meters to reach a HR of 166 and spent 64 percent of that rep at or above 166. Compared to 40 percent during 800s at 5K pace.

Run mile repeats at 5K pace and you'll spend a huge percentage of training time at your 5K HR goals, and be forced to make improvements to your running efficiency to achieve these sessions.

The lower heartrate in the last column is probably a reflection of our hamster concentrating on his running efficiency while dealing with his fatigue, and perhaps because he had sweated off some of his over-hydration, so he was at ideal running weight for this final 5:53 of running at 5K pace.

You'll spend an even greater percentage of your time at 5K HR if you add a fifth lap to get 2,000 meter repeats! The fifth lap can feel a little gruesome though, so try to run it with company.

Lets see how much of your training is likely to be at ideal **anaerobic threshold HR** (90 % of max HR) while running 1,200s with short rests. Our athlete runs 6 x 1,200 on a nearly straight section of grass and no undulations. Using a two minute rest, (200 meters of mostly jogging…HR down to 120) he averages 4.37 per repeat (slowest first at 4.40; fastest 4.35 in the middle and a 4.39 finish). His maximum HR is 180; a seasoned runner of several decades, his goal HR for 15K pace is 162.

Repeat #	1	2	3	4	5	6
Point at which						
HR reached 162 at	900	550	350	250	200	150 meters
HR at 400	149	157	162	163	164	163
HR at 800	159	163	164	163	162	162
HR at 1,200	163	164	164	164	163	163

percentage of time the heart was at						
15K intensity	25	54	62	80	83	87 %

* The highest HR this day was actually 165, (950 meters into the 3rd rep) which is 10K intensity, and not the goal of his session. He reduced pace to get back to a 164 HR.
* The relatively slow first repeat contributed to only 25 percent of it being at 15K HR goals. However, the entire three quarters of a mile were at his 15K speed for the year, and the sensible start set up a pleasurable session.
* The 90 % level took 550 meters for the second repeat, with 54 % of his repetition at goal HR, and over three-quarters was above 85 % of max HR (threshold level for many people).
* As the session progressed, a pleasant fatigue set in and 90 % of max HR was achieved very early in each repeat, giving him 83 % of his time, or eleven and a quarter minutes at his 15K goal HR during the last three repeats.
* While he had the legs to do at least one more repeat, he saved himself for his long run the next day.
* He eased the pace just a little for the last two repeats to stop himself hitting 10K HR intensity.

How can we improve his anaerobic threshold?

1. Have him run another 4.5 mile threshold session every 4 to 5 days for 6 to 8 weeks.
2. Match each threshold session with short effort fartlek or 5K pace running alternating with hills.
3. Include tempo runs and longer repeats. When he does this session again, consider:

4. Running the first rep a bit faster and taking a one minute rest before the second repeat, which should get him to a 162 HR by perhaps 600 and 400 meters during those repeats, which would result in an additional 450 meters at a HR of 162. Then use 2 minutes rests so that:
5. He can add an additional repeat once a month. Or,
6. Increase length of repeats to one mile, which would give him an additional 92 seconds at his threshold HR on all six repeats. This would take his current 47 % at goal HR during the first three repeats to 62 %. In total, he would get an additional 1.5 miles or over 9 minutes at goal HR.
7. Ask him to do a maximum HR test to make sure his max HR has not dropped to 178. If his max HR is 178, the training time at 164 HR would be in his 10K range. While that would be a very nice session, unless he can race 15K at this intensity, it is too harsh for anaerobic threshold training. (Note: If he is training in his 10K range he will obviously not be able to race a 15K at that pace!)

The last four pages came from:

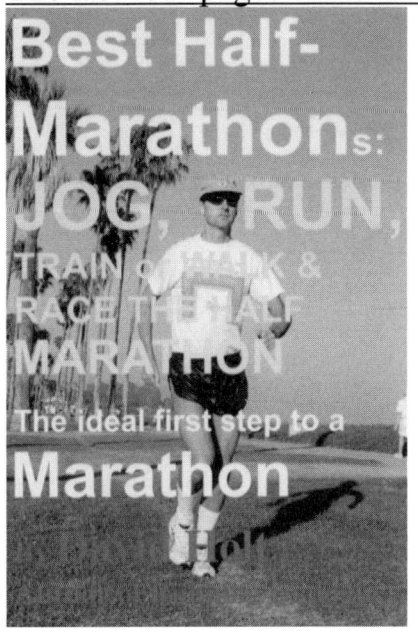

Best Half-Marathons: *Jog, Run, Train or Walk & Race the Half Marathon.* 224 pages. ISBN # 0-9658897-6-9 $17.95. Graduate from 5K training with a year at the half-marathon, which will lay the foundation for marathon training or make you stronger for the 5K and 10K. Schedules for half marathon to 20 mile racing. Includes 10 to 50 week programs with practice races and a monthly restive week, motivation and the scientific training techniques.

INDEX

THE AUTHOR

David Holt's 15:18 for the 5K came just after his 30th birthday...the result of over a decade of competent and varied training and minimal talent.

Registered Nurse David has <u>run</u> with many international class runners, has <u>trained</u> with dozens of competent club runners, and run & trained with hundreds of recreational runners (some of whom called themselves joggers).

The English club system helped David to 31:16 for 10,000 meters (5:02 per mile) and 67:52 for the 20K.

In his third decade of competitive running, David also cross trains with biking, elliptical training, pool running, swimming and weight training. Note that they were listed alphabetically!

David has sold articles to Runner's World and Running Times. His printed books are *Running Dialogue, 10K & 5K Running, Training & Racing, Best Half-Marathons* and *Best Marathons. 5K Fitness Run* is available on paper or in e-book format.

Holt's other e-books include:

Best Half Marathons: Jog, Run, Train or Walk & Race the Half Marathon is also available as an e-book.

Best Marathons: Jog, Run, Train or Walk & Race Fast Marathons.

401 Injury Prevention and Treatment tips to Walk, Jog, Run or Train 6 days a week.

10K & 5K Running: Jog, Run and Train to Race 5K, 10K to 10 Miles (An e-book version of the printed 10K & 5K Running)

301 Balanced Eating & Nutrition Tips: Don't Diet for Exercise & Health.

Other E-books available soon will be:

Athletic Cross Training for Runners & Triathletes: Pool run, weight or elliptical train, bike & walk or jog to fitness. Hint: You already own half of this cross training book.

5K Fitness Walk, Jog or Run for Health: Decrease your death risk from over 20 diseases and conditions.

50 runs to your 10K: 10 week program to jog, train & race a 10K. Buying options for printed copies of David Holt's running books are on page 240.

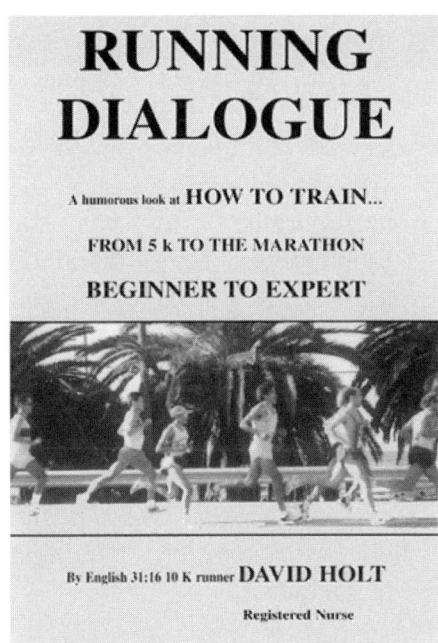

Running Dialogue, 5K to the Marathon, 280 pages ISBN # 0-9658897-4-2 is $17.95. The Ideal first book for beginners or as an addition to your running book library. Includes advice for beginning a running program, making better use of your exercise time with hill training, anaerobic threshold and sane Interval running, plus humor, injury and nutrition advice and how to prepare for racing at 5K to the marathon.

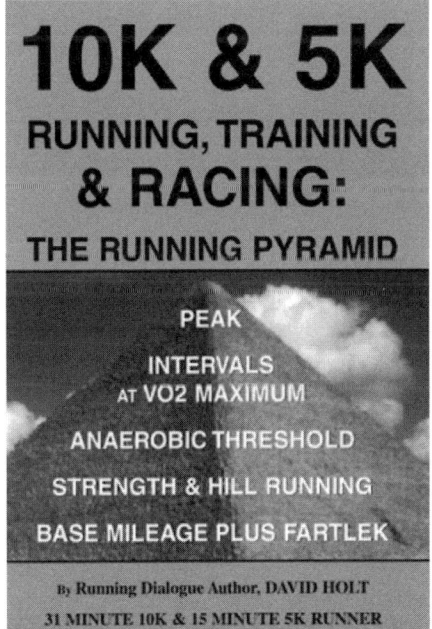

10K & 5K Running, Training & Racing: The Running Pyramid, 180 pages ISBN # 0-9658897-1-8 is $17.95. Five training phases for 5K to 10K racing. Low intensity 20 mile per week runners enjoy the science and running techniques as much as the 60 mile per week runners. Each runner has a special section. Includes a book summary just before each training schedule for easy reference.

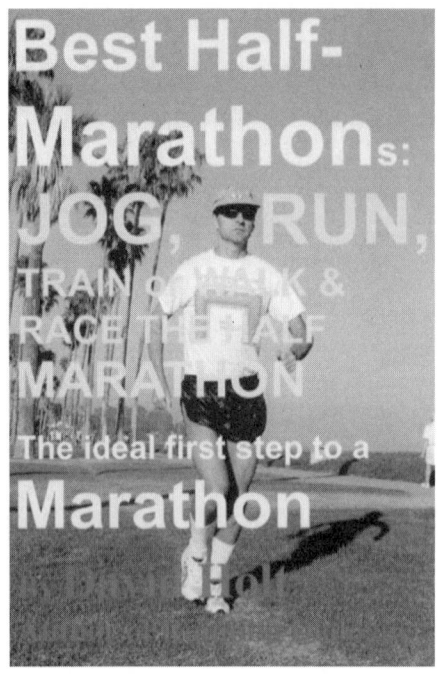

Best Half-Marathons*:* *Jog, Run, Train or Walk & Race the Half Marathon.* 224 pages. ISBN # 0-9658897-6-9 $17.95. Graduate from 5K & 10K training with a year at the half-marathon to lay the foundation for marathon training or to make yourself stronger for the 5K & 10K. Schedules for half marathon to 20 mile racing. Includes 10 to 50 week programs with practice races and a monthly restive week, motivation and the scientific training techniques.

E-books have to be ordered from online bookstores.

David Holt is also at http://www.runningbook.com

For your buying convenience, David Holt's web site has links to Amazon.com for all of his books.

Order Form: For books on paper
Send checks to David Holt,   PO Box 543
                 Goleta, CA 93116

Include Name and address you wish the book(s) to be sent to.

Pay $16.00 for the first book and $14.00 per copy for additional books. Order any combination to get the discount. Shipping and sales tax is included.

Tell me the titles and quantities of the books that you require.